DERMABRASION
AND
CHEMICAL PEEL

Published Volumes

Proportions of the Aesthetic Face
Powell and Humphreys

Facial Reconstruction with Local and Regional Flaps
Becker

Rhinoplasty: Emphasizing the External Approach
Anderson and Ries

Surgery of the Mandible
Bailey and Holt

Lasers in Skin Disease
Wheeland

Forthcoming Volumes

Facial Plastic Surgery in the Asian
McCurdy

Hair Rejuvenation
Fleming and Mayer

Microsurgical Reconstruction of the Head and Neck
Panje and Moran

Rhinoplasty
Simons

The American Academy of Facial Plastic and Reconstructive Surgery

Series Editor: James D. Smith, M.D.

DERMABRASION AND CHEMICAL PEEL

A Guide for Facial Plastic Surgeons

E. Gaylon McCollough, M.D., F.A.C.S.
President and Founder
McCollough International Facial Plastic Surgeons

Clinical Professor, Department of Surgery, Otolaryngology
University of Alabama — Birmingham

Phillip Royal Langsdon, M.D.
Langsdon Facial Plastic Surgery
Memphis, Tennessee

Clinical Assistant Professor of Dermatologic Surgery
Department of Medicine, Division of Dermatology
University of Tennessee — Memphis

1988
Thieme Medical Publishers, Inc., New York
Georg Thieme Verlag, Stuttgart · New York

Thieme Medical Publishers, Inc.
381 Park Avenue South
New York, New York 10016

Series sponsored by the Educational Committee of The Ameri-can Academy of Facial Plastic and Reconstructive Surgery.

DERMABRASION AND CHEMICAL PEEL
E. Gaylon McCollough and Phillip Royal Langsdon

Library of Congress Cataloging-in-Publication Data

McCollough, E. Gaylon.
  Dermabrasion and chemical peel.

  (The American Academy of Facial Plastic and
Reconstructive Surgery)
  Bibliography: p.
  Includes index.
  1. Dermabrasion. 2. Chemical peel. 3. Face—
Surgery. 4. Surgery, Plastic. I. Langsdon, Phillip R.
II. Title. III. Series: The American Academy of Facial
Plastic and Reconstructive Surgery (Series) [DNLM:
1. Chemexfoliation—adverse effects. 2. Chemexfoliation
—methods. 3. Dermabrasion—adverse effects. 4. Derma-
brasion—methods. 5. Face—surgery. 6. Surgery,
Plastic. WE 705 M4777d]
RD523.M39 1988   617′.520592   88-24971
ISBN 0-86577-284-3

Printed in the United States of America.

TMP ISBN 0-86577-284-3
GTV ISBN 3-13-729001-5

TMP (series) 0-86577-137-5
GTV (series) 3-13-656501-0

Important Note: Medicine is an ever-changing science. Research and clinical experience are continually broadening our knowledge, in particular our knowledge of proper treatment and drug therapy. Insofar as this book mentions any dosage or application, readers may rest assured that the authors, editors, and publishers have made every effort to ensure that such references are strictly in accordance with the state of knowledge at the time of production of the book. Nevertheless, every user is requested to carefully examine the manufacturers' leaflets accompanying each drug to check on his own responsibility whether the dosage schedules recommended therein or the contraindications stated by the manufacturers differ from the statements made in the present book. Such examination is particularly important with drugs that are either rarely used or have been newly released on the market.

Some of the product names, patents and registered designs referred to in this book are in fact registered trademarks or proprietary names even though specific reference to this fact is not always made in the text. Therefore, the appearance of a name without designation as proprietary is not to be construed as a representation by the publisher that it is in the public domain.

1 2 3 4 5 6 7 8 9 10

Contents

Preface

Increasing numbers of men and women are seeking improvement in their appearance. Approximately 600,000 Americans undergo cosmetic surgery each year. A cosmetic or reconstructive surgical procedure often may not yield the optimum result due to associated wrinkling, scarring, or pigmentation of the facial skin. Dermabrasion and chemical peel are techniques that facial plastic surgeons can add to their armamentarium to improve the quality and texture of a patient's skin. Since both procedures involve the removal of the "damaged" epidermis and superficial layers of the dermis, new skin regeneration generally leaves the patient with more youthful-looking skin.

The appearance of surgical simplicity should not be misinterpreted. Chemical peel and dermabrasion are surgical procedures; therefore, the necessary precautions must be exercised. Both procedures can achieve pleasing results, but each could be associated with unwarranted complications, ranging from aberrations of skin pigment and scarring to even death.

It is the intention of the authors for this monograph to serve as a guideline to obtaining predictable results with the use of dermabrasion and chemical peel. On the other hand, there is no substitute for experience and training at centers where large volumes of these procedures are performed.

As one learns new surgical procedures, he or she should proceed with caution. The slightest variation in technique may result in an undesirable outcome. For this reason it may be wise to observe a facial plastic surgeon who is expertly proficient in a given procedure and adopt his or her protocol.

There are numerous similarities and dissimilarities in the two procedures with regard to technique and clinical application. Each procedure will be reviewed with respect to indications, post-operative care, complications, and results. Hopefully, this compendium shall serve as a reference for the facial plastic surgeon treating facial skin irregularities and rhytids.

THE GREAT DEBATE: DERMABRASION VERSUS CHEMICAL PEEL

A continuing debate exists over which procedure—dermabrasion or chemical peel—is superior for treating rhytids, scars, sun-damaged skin, and pigmentation problems. There is probably no right or wrong answer. The results of either procedure depends upon a number of variables, ranging from the skill of the surgeon to the pathologic condition being treated.

It is difficult to make a comparison between the results of dermabrasion and chemical peel because of the variables introduced by the individual surgeon. For example, dermabrasion may be performed with or without freezing the skin. The depth of the freeze and number of times the area is refrozen introduce differing degrees of tissue insult. The actual procedure may be performed with many different types of instrumentation, ranging from wire brushes to diamond fraises and even standard hardware sandpaper. The depth of dermabrasion varies among surgeons, and from one area of the face to another.

Post-operative care may affect the final result. Maibach and Rovee have demonstrated that abraded wounds allowed to dry and form a crust heal more slowly and at a deeper level than wounds treated with the moist-dressing technique.

One can surmise, therefore, that it is not the term given to the procedure that should be used for comparison purposes; all of the variables just mentioned must be considered in any attempt to compare dermabrasion to any other procedure.

Chemical peel or chemexfoliation is the term given to a procedure in which any mixture of chemicals is applied to the skin's surface, thereby producing tissue insult and an inflammatory reaction.

Many different chemical formulas have been used in an attempt to cause varying amounts of the epidermis and dermis to slough, so that "new" skin, with a more youthful histologic morphology, might replace the wrinkled or weathered appearance of the aging skin.

Chemical formulas include a number of materials: 1) resorcinol or retinoic acid, which produces a mild irritation to the superficial layers with some temporary and minimal improvement; 2) trichloroacetic acid (TCA), with different concentrations that, by design, produce varying degrees of tissue destruction and unpredictable results; and 3) phenol formulas, which produce greater degrees of second-degree insult. In the experience of the authors, the formula, containing phenol, croton oil, liquid soap, and water, seems to afford the most dramatic and predictable method for treating the pathologic conditions indicated for chemical peel (see Part Two's introductory section).

Even with the identical formula, the results of chemical peel will vary, depending upon a number of factors.

If the facial plastic surgeon fails to remove all oils from the skin surface, the exfoliant will not penetrate evenly or to the desired depth. Scrubbing the facial skin with an abrasive gauze saturated with acetone provides the best preparation. The amount of solution applied to each region will also determine the depth of tissue insult.

Much debate exists over immediate occlusion with waterproof dressings, performed immediately after the solution is applied to produce greater penetration of the exfoliant.

The senior author has performed this procedure with and without taping. It has been surmised that a greater degree of maceration is produced by water- and airtight occlusion, but the tissue insult produced by the additional maceration can be produced by more vigorous "scrubbing" with acetone before exfoliant application and by the application of greater amounts of the exfoliant during the procedure.

The authors' experiences validate the conclusions of Maibach and Rovee in that crust formation over the surface of abraded or exfoliated wounds delays healing by approximately 40 to 50%. The additional insult to the papillary dermis produced by the inflammatory reaction at the base of the crust can also be offset by a proper acetone-abrasive preparation and by slightly more exfoliant applied to the treated areas.

One can quickly realize that a number of variables determine the end result of both chemical peel and dermabrasion. Not only is it difficult to compare chemical peel to dermabrasion, but it is also difficult to compare one facial plastic surgeon's dermabrasion or chemical peel technique to another's.

Facial plastic surgeons must therefore take the available information and develop a technique that works best for them. The surgeon will then possess the flexibility to use any of the variables at his or her disposal to provide *each* patient with the best result achievable in a specific situation.

The material presented in this book represents the opinions and experiences of the authors, and it is intended to serve as a guideline for obtaining more predictable results with both dermabrasion and chemexfoliation (chemical peel).

The authors hope that the contents of this book shall provide the foundation for the surgeon-artist to practice his or her profession with greater insight and improved skills.

E. Gaylon McCollough
Phillip Royal Langsdon

Introduction

An introduction to skin anatomy and wound healing characteristics is important to any surgeon performing facial plastic surgery. Regional variations exist in the skin anatomy. However, the basic structure is the same all over the body. Nerves, capillaries, sweat glands, sebaceous glands, hair follicles, keratin content, and melanocytes are present in varying percentages in the different anatomic regions.

The outer epidermis and inner dermis constitute the two major layers of skin (Fig. 1). The epidermis is composed of a stratum corneum, stratum lucidum, stratum granulosum, stratum spinosum, and stratum germinativum. The stratum corneum is replaced every 14 days. It takes about the same amount of time for a cell produced on the basal layer to reach the stratum corneum. Melanin is produced by the melanocytes contained within the basal cell layer. Skin color is determined by its thickness and vascularity, as well as by its melanin content (Figs. 2, 3).

The dermis is composed of a superficial papillary layer and a deeper, tougher reticular layer. The reticular layer is responsible for the strength of the skin. The dermis contains numerous blood vessels and nerves that course through small evaginations projecting into the epidermis (dermal papillae). In 1 mm² of skin, there might be as many as 100 papillae. The dermis is composed of collagen, ground substance, reticular fibers, elastic fibers, and mucopolysaccharides. Fibroblasts, mast cells, and histiocytes are also found in this layer.

The skin appendages, such as hair, sweat glands, and sebaceous glands, are embryologically derived from the epidermis. The ability of the skin to regenerate is directly related to the amount of normal adnexae (pilosebaceous apparatus and sweat glands [Fig. 4]). The skin of different regions of the body contain varying quantities of adnexae. Facial skin, for example, is rich in dermal adnexa compared to skin of the inner aspect of the arm. Therefore, if done properly, dermabrasion may be performed on the face without frequent complications because of the regenerative properties of the skin. On the other hand, one could expect slower healing and a higher incidence of complications if the same procedure is performed on the arm.

When considering the head and neck region, it must be understood that the base of the neck, suprasternal area, and eyelids are regions covered by thin skin containing relatively sparse adnexa. These areas, therefore, are more susceptible to hypertrophic scar formation due to the inadequate regenerative capacity of the thin skin via its lack of dermal appendages. To obtain satisfactory results with either dermabrasion or

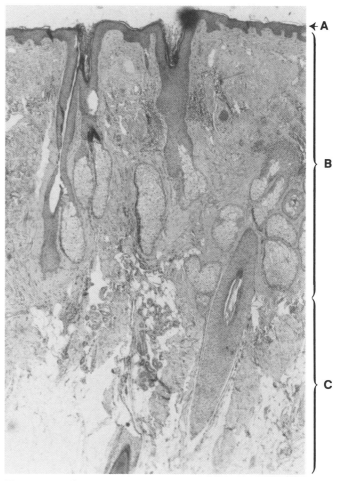

Figure 1. Cross-section of facial skin showing epidermis (A), dermis (B), and subcutaneous layers (C). Note plentiful hair follicles, sebaceous glands, and eccrine sweat glands. (Photo courtesy of Edwin A. Raines, M.D., Memphis, Tennessee.)

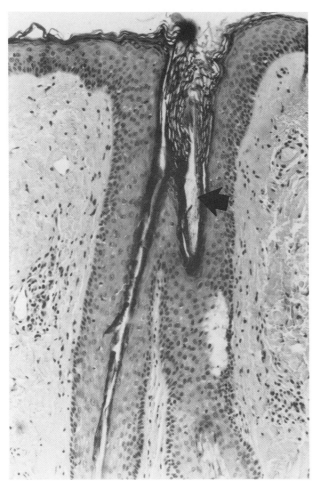

Figure 2. Cross-section of facial skin. Note epidermis cell layers. Also note dermal matrix containing small blood vessels and follicular infundibulum (see arrow). (Photo courtesy of Edwin A. Raines, M.D., Memphis, Tennessee.)

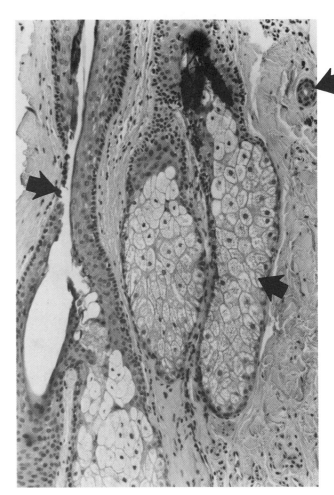

Figure 4. Cross section of facial skin. Note eccrine sweat gland (top right), sebaceous glands (lower right), and isthmus of hair follicle (left). (Photo courtesy of Edwin A. Raines, M.D., Memphis, Tennessee.)

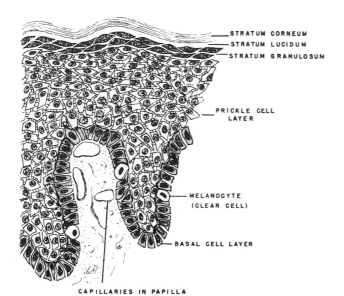

STRATUM CORNEUM
STRATUM LUCIDUM
STRATUM GRANULOSUM

PRICKLE CELL LAYER

MELANOCYTE (CLEAR CELL)

BASAL CELL LAYER

CAPILLARIES IN PAPILLA

Figure 3. Cross-section of epidermis. (From Noojin RO [ed]: *Dermatology for Students.* Springfield, Illinois, Charles C. Thomas, 1961, p. 4.)

chemical peel, the facial plastic surgeon must remove adequate amounts of epidermis and perform surgery in the dermis. If the surgical insult is extended below the deeper layers of the dermis, scar formation could occur. If the surgical insult is extended no deeper than the mid-dermis, adequate regeneration will occur, as long as dermal adnexae are plentiful. With adequate post-operative care, the epidermal regeneration process should be evident in about five days. New collagen formation within the dermis will occur for a period after this initial process of epidermal healing. Although the epidermis generally regenerates to its original thickness, dermal healing is somewhat delayed, and may never reach the original thickness.

WOUND HEALING

In controlled animal studies, the healing process post-injury begins with some initial bleeding, which normally coagulates and becomes a crust within 24 hours if undisturbed. The crust may remain for as long as three weeks before it is shed.

The regeneration process begins with epithelial formation. Migration occurs first from the wound margin, and second from the pilosebaceous apparatus. This epithelial regeneration begins as early as 18 to 24 hours post-injury, and may be complete after seven days.

Vascular dilatation occurs, and the tiny vessels become filled with leukocytes. Swelling in the wound develops as the cells and fluid escape the vascular channels.

By day seven, fibroblasts appear, and the undersurface of the new epidermis develops ridges. Collagen proliferation is detectable by day nine. By day 15, dermal contraction is evident, and the initial healing is completed by day 40.

Several factors may be responsible for a delay in the healing process. For example, an inadequate vascular supply may impede the process by denying some of the regenerative cells, nutrients, and fluids free access to the healing area. An insufficient amount of dermal appendages, which are essential to epithelial regeneration, can also delay healing. An important consideration is the amount of crusting that forms on the exposed (uncovered) wound surface. The dry crust scab forces epithelial migration to tunnel beneath the crust. This crust may serve as a mechanical barrier to the regenerative process. Maibach and Rovee[1] have shown that the healing process occurs more rapidly over a moist surface covered with a lubricant or nonadherent dressing. The covered surface prevents crust formation and maintains a fluid medium. Epithelial migration may be completed within 24 hours in a moist human wound. The crusted wound, on the other hand, may require two or three days. Because epithelial migration would proceed deeply to the plain of crusting, the uncovered wound could result in a depressed skin surface after healing is completed. A covered wound, which maintains a fluid medium, allows epithelial regeneration to occur with less resistance and at a more rapid rate. The following discussions of dermabrasion and chemical peel describe a technique of post-operative management employing the "moist surface" philosophy. The authors have found

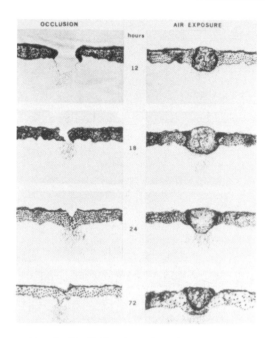

Figure 5. Epithelialization in air-exposed or occluded incisions. Completion of epithelialization occurs at 18 to 24 hours under occlusion and at two to three days in air exposure. There is no scab formation in occluded incisions and no apparent tissue loss through dehydration. Note the plane of new epidermis in air-exposed incisions at 72 hours. (From Winter GD: Epidermal regeneration studied in the domestic pig; and Rovee DT, et al: Effect of local wound environment on epidermal healing. In Maibach HI, Rovee DT [eds]: *Epidermal Wound Healing.* Chicago, Yearbook Medical Publishers, 1972.)

that wounds heal much more quickly and result in more comfort to the patient during the healing process (Fig. 5).

After the initial phase of wound healing, the regenerative process continues for a period of time. In some cases, this maturation phase may be complete after six months, or it can take as long as 18 months in younger patients. During this period, the rejuvenated collagen fibers of the dermis are realigned into the more parallel pattern of youthful skin. The auxilliary capillaries of healing regress. The wound softens, flattens, and becomes lighter in color.

PART ONE

DERMABRASION

INTRODUCTION

Dermabrasion is generally performed when it is desirable to remove the epidermis and superficial layers of the dermis in order to smooth irregularities and camouflage scarring. It has been used, at times, as a therapeutic modality to treat cystic acne, particularly when conventional medical treatments have proven unsuccessful. The indications for dermabrasion are listed in Table 1.

INSTRUMENTATION

Numerous methods are used to remove the superficial layer of skin through dermabrading. Originally, carpenter sandpaper was employed to hand plane the skin to remove irregularities. Later, the idea of a motor-driven instrument was developed to abrade the skin. Some surgeons tried dental drill units, consisting of a motor with pulleys and belts to drive the handpiece. Early on, sandpaper discs on a bit were attached to the dental unit.

Special dermabrading units have been developed that make dental instruments obsolete. The first units relied upon the use of a motor-driven cable. These instruments were complicated by the fact that the cables could not be bent in acute angles, and careful attention had to be paid that the cables were relatively straight.

Air-driven units have also been used by some operators. The authors prefer the Bell International Hand Engine, which rotates at 600 to 20,000 rpm. A slightly more powerful unit rotating at 1,500 to 35,000 rpm is also available (Fig. 6).

In the authors' experience, freezing the skin has been a great aid to dermabrasion via fixing the

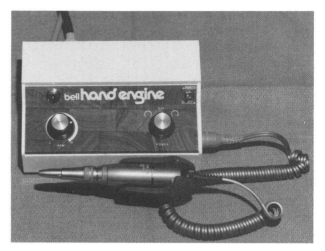

Figure 6. Hand engine with foot pedal control and variable speed (electric motor).

skin into an iceball so that it would not move under the rapidly turning handpiece. Originally, ethyl chloride spray was used for freezing, but this agent was found to be both toxic and flammable. Freon (di-chloro-tetra-floro-ethane) is nonflammable, odorless, and nontoxic. Currently, it is the agent most commonly used (Fig. 7).

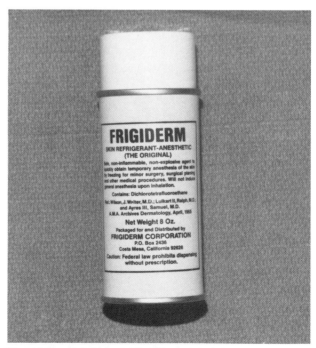

Figure 7. Frigiderm (di-chloro-tetra-floro-ethane) is nonflammable, odorless, and nontoxic.

Table 1. Indications for Dermabrasion

Acne scarring
Active acne (not responsive to medical therapy)
Nasal rhinophyma
Traumatic or surgical scarring
Tattoos
Lentigenes
Facial rhytids
Keratoses (seborrheic or actinic)

GOALS OF DERMABRASION

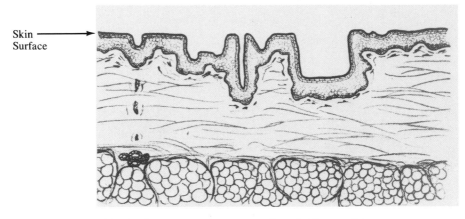

Skin Surface →

This drawing represents a cross-section of skin containing acne scars. The scars may vary in depth, width and configuration. Some are very deep, penetrating far down into the dermis.

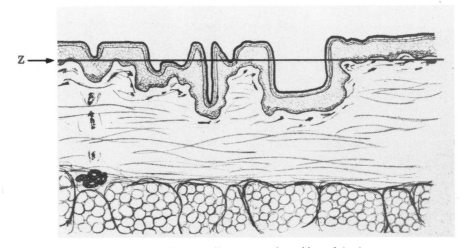

Z →

Dermabrasion (at level Z) generally removes the epidermal (top) layer of skin. Many of the more superficial scars may be completely eliminated, and the scars of intermediate depth improved; but the deeper ones are only slightly better.

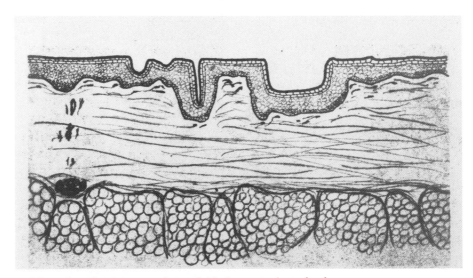

After a dermabrasion, a new layer of skin forms at a lower level.

From *Plastic Surgery: Face, Head, and Neck* by E. G. McCollough. Ebsco Media, Birmingham, AL, 1984.

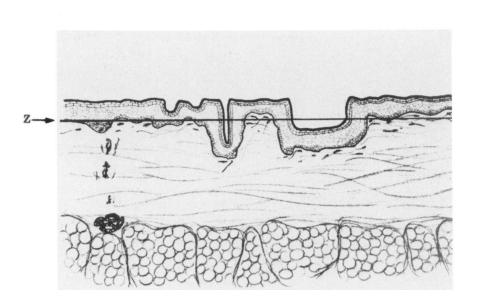

Often a second dermabrasion (at level Z) can be performed within another 6 to 12 months.

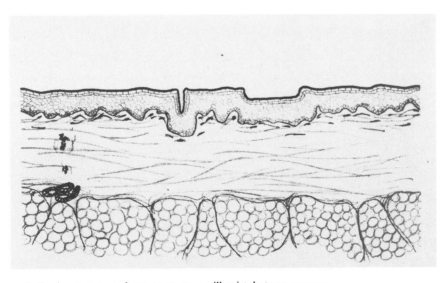

Following two procedures, some scars still exist; but one may see improvement in the overall texture and consistency of the skin.

Several types of dermabrasion tips are available, including wire brushes, diamond fraises, and serrated stainless steel wheels. They come in a variety of sizes and shapes. In most instances, the authors prefer the wire brush, measuring 17 mm in diameter and 6 mm in width. Occasionally, in the periorbital areas and around the nasal alar creases, we use small, rounded diamond burs (Fig. 8).

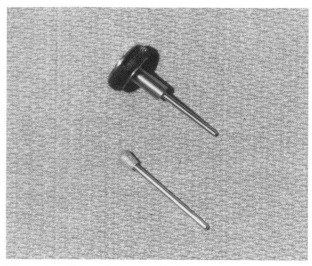

Figure 8.   17 mm × 6 mm wire brush and pear-shaped diamond fraise.

1   Patient Selection

Dermabrasion is most often performed to obtain improvement in skin that has been scarred due to chronic acne. Almost all acne scarring can be somewhat improved with a properly performed dermabrasion procedure. The degree of improvement, however, is directly related to the type and severity of scarring.

ACNE SCARRING

Severe scarring that contains bridges and tunnels often requires cold knife planing of the surface mounds to expose the underlying tissues. One problem often encountered with this condition is that after the superficial knife planing, scarring may seem worse when, in reality, the scarring was simply covered by superficial skin bridges. Several dermabrasion procedures spaced 6 to 12 months apart may be needed to obtain maximum improvement with this type of problem (Figs. 9a–c).

The more superficial acne scars often respond best to dermabrasion. Here, also, more than one procedure may be required to achieve the best possible result (Figs. 10a–d).

Deep scars complicated by surrounding skin contractions are most commonly seen in the patient with cystic acne. This condition does not respond as well as the more superficially located, crater-like lesions and requires multiple procedures to obtain improvement (Fig. 11).

The authors have noticed an improvement in both the degree and severity of active acne lesions after patients have undergone a dermabrasion procedure for old scars. It could be that dermabrasion is the ultimate skin cleansing procedure. The fact that the acne has improved is probably related to the opening of the pilosebaceous apparatus for better drainage (Fig. 12).

ACTIVE ACNE

If a patient has active acne when a dermabrasion procedure is performed, he or she should be informed that dermabrasion will not cure the disease process, but may *improve* the condition, at least for a period of time. Most patients usually require continued medical treatment. Repeated dermabrasion procedures may be required to improve severely scarred skin or skin with an irregular surface.

NASAL RHINOPHYMA

Patients with nasal rhinophyma (acne rosacea) can often obtain dramatic improvement from removal of the thick sebaceous epithelium. Superficial planing with cold or hot knife blades may often be required to first

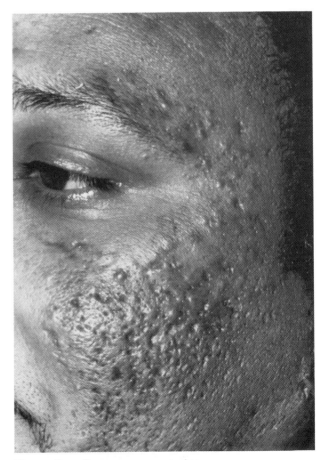

Figure 9a.   Severe acne scarring.

7

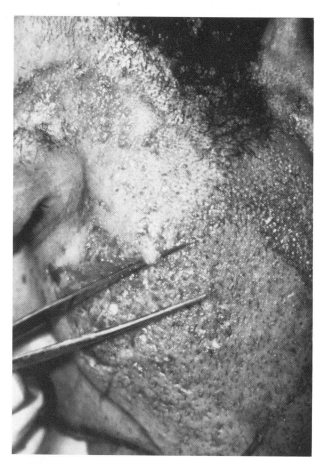

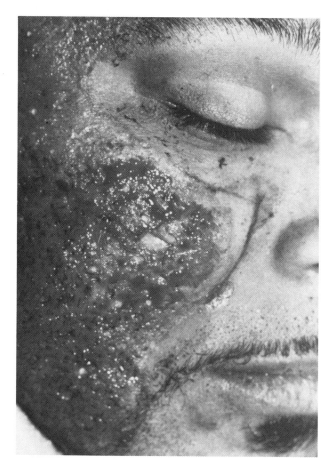

Figure 9b. After the superficial layers are removed, skin bridges and tunnels appear. Forceps are deep to scar tissue bridge.

Figure 9c. Deep scar pits and cysts may be uncovered.

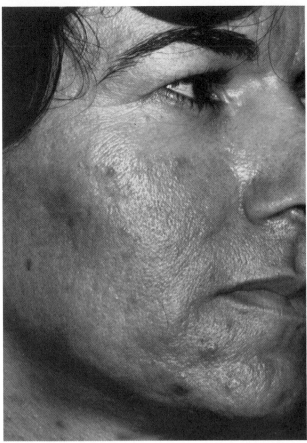

Figure 10a. Acne scarring in noncystic acne (right oblique view).

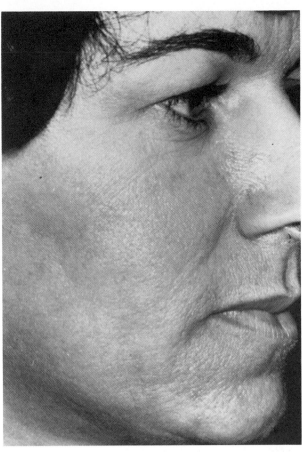

Figure 10c. After one dermabrasion (right oblique view).

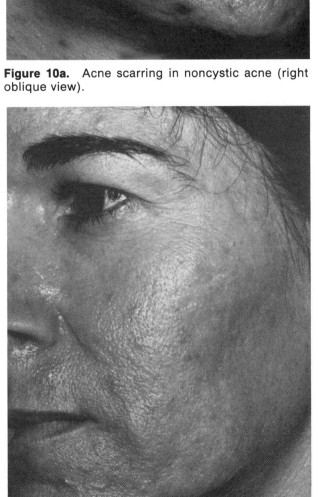

Figure 10b. Acne scarring in noncystic acne (left oblique view).

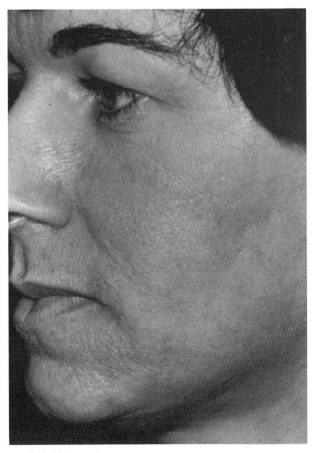

Figure 10d. After one dermabrasion (left oblique view).

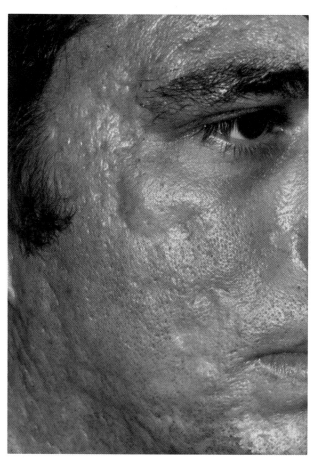

Figure 11a.   Deep acne scarring.

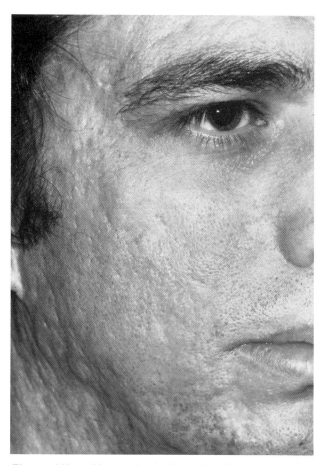

Figure 11b.   After a single dermabrasion, this patient experienced some overall improvement. Deep scars cannot be totally removed.

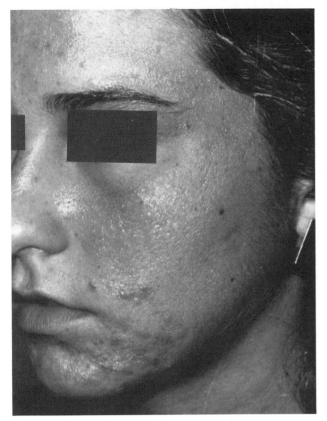

Figure 12a. Active acne (left oblique view).

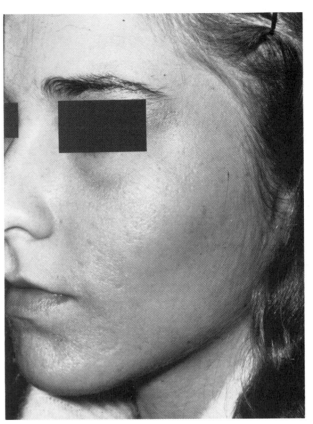

Figure 12c. Seven months post-dermabrasion (left oblique view).

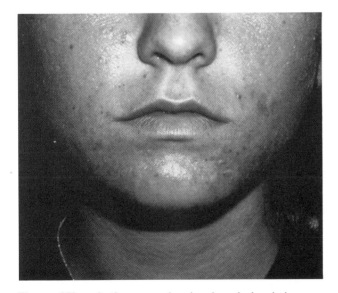

Figure 12b. Active acne (perioral and cheeks).

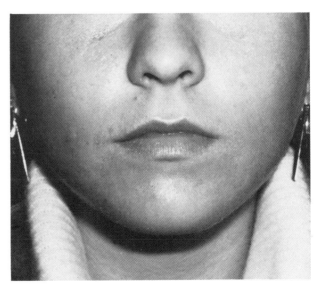

Figure 12d. Seven months post-dermabrasion (perioral and cheeks).

shave the tissues down to the desired level. The dermabrader device can be used to accurately contour the nose into its final shape, while removing the unwanted cutaneous tissue. As with any other region requiring dermabrasion, care must be taken to remove tissue to about the mid-dermal level. Removal of the thick epidermal skin with a knife blade often allows one to more carefully observe the depth as the dermis is approached during a dermabrasion procedure. Stabilization of the nasal tip is a technical problem encountered while dermabrading the nose. Freezing is often required to fix the tissues, so that the tip may be more easily and accurately sculpted (Fig. 13).

TRAUMATIC OR SURGICAL SCARRING

Other types of scarring, due to trauma or surgical incisions, may be improved by dermabrasion. Scars wider than 0.5 cm, however, are best excised and allowed to heal for a period of six months, or until the scars are mature before dermabrasion surgery is attempted. At times, scars may need to be dermabraded two to three times to achieve the desired results. The best results are generally obtained when a scar is localized and not attached to the underlying tissues. Superficial scarring often responds well to dermabrasion. When elevated tissues surrounding scars are planed (as one

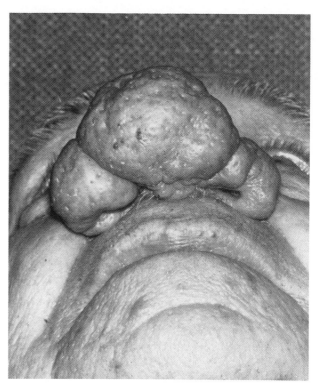

Figure 13b. Rhinophyma (base view).

would sand down a piece of wood containing multiple scratches), a smoother surface reduces shadows from certain types of light and provides a more pleasing appearance (Fig. 14).

Elevated scars that are mature and not hypertrophic can be planed down to the level of the surrounding skin. In this situation, it is best to dermabrade the scar down to a level just below the surface of the

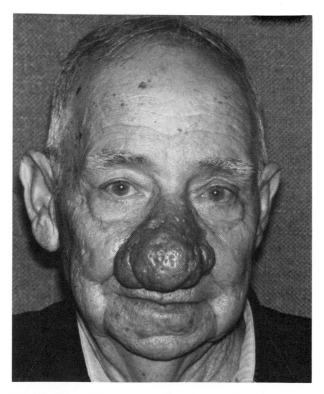

Figure 13a. Rhinophyma (frontal view).

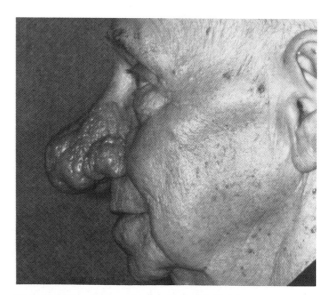

Figure 13c. Rhmophyma (lateral view).

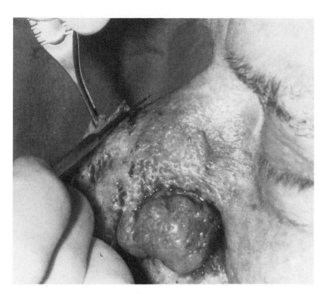

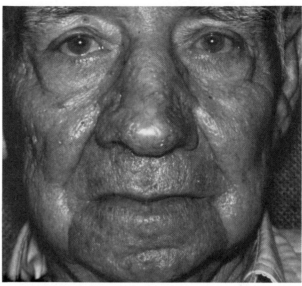

Figure 13f. After knife planing and dermabrasion (frontal view).

Figure 13d. Knife planing, dorsal tip region. Knife planing often is used to shave the excess tissues down to a level more desirable for dermabrasion.

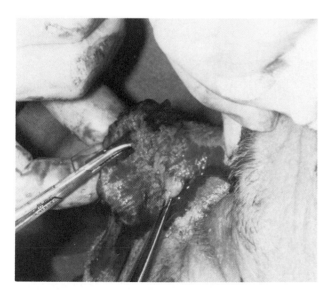

Figure 13e. Knife planing, lateral nose.

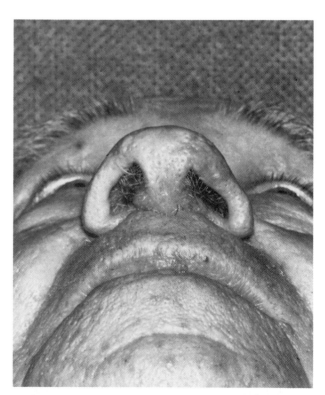

Figure 13g. After knife planing and dermabrasion (base view).

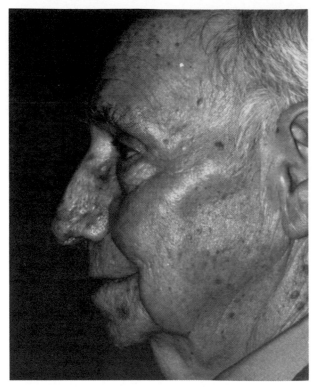

Figure 13h. After knife planing and dermabrasion (lateral view).

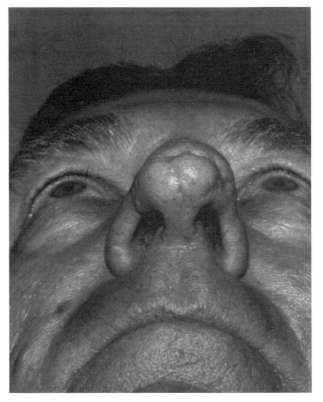

Figure 14b. Base view.

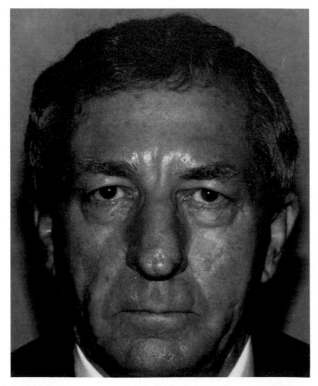

Figure 14a. Hypertrophic sebaceous nasal tissue accentuates this old scar (frontal view).

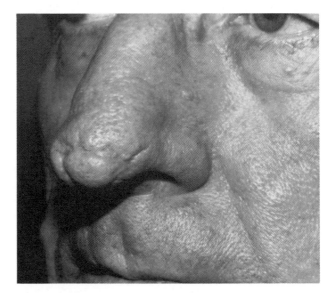

Figure 14c. Left oblique view.

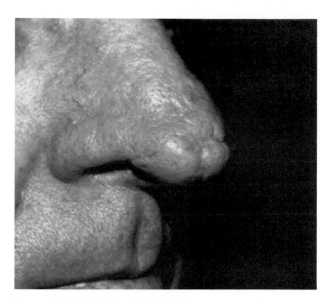

Figure 14d. Right oblique view.

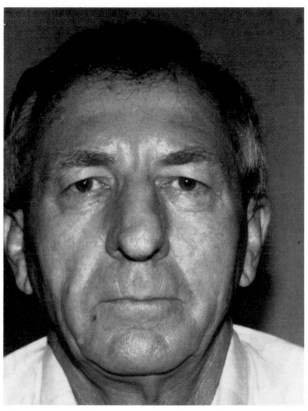

Figure 14f. After dermabrasion, sebaceous tissue now level with scar (frontal view).

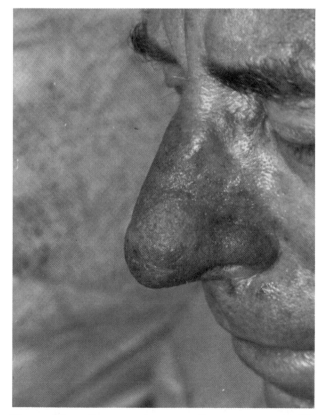

Figure 14e. Excess sebaceous tissue removed with wire brush; tissue now level with scar.

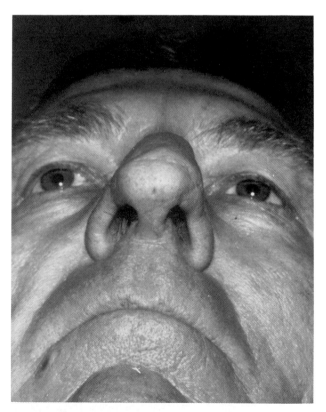

Figure 14g. After dermabrasion, sebaceous tissue now level with scar (base view).

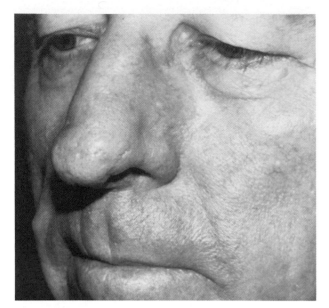

Figure 14h. After dermabrasion, sebaceous tissue now level with scar (left oblique view).

surrounding skin for the new tissues to bridge the defect during the regenerative process.

Surgical excisional techniques before a dermabrasion procedure are usually recommended for scars that are too wide, too deep, longer than 1 inch, cross-natural creases or facial contour lines, elevated above the adjacent skin, depressed below the adjacent skin, or a different color than adjacent tissues (Figs. 15 to 19).

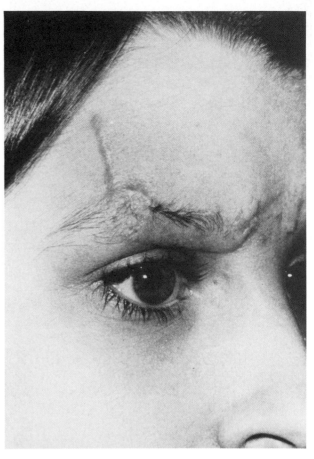

Figure 15a. Forehead, brow, and eyelid scarring.

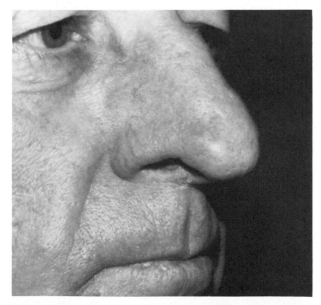

Figure 14i. After dermabrasion, sebaceous tissue now level with scar (right oblique view).

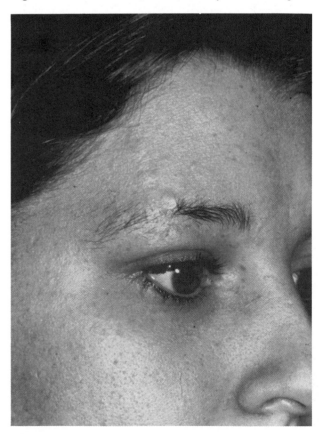

Figure 15b. Post-operative scar revision.

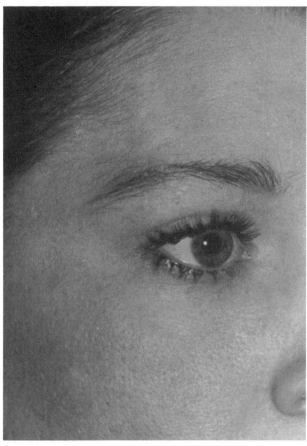

Figure 15c. Post-operative scar revision and dermabrasion.

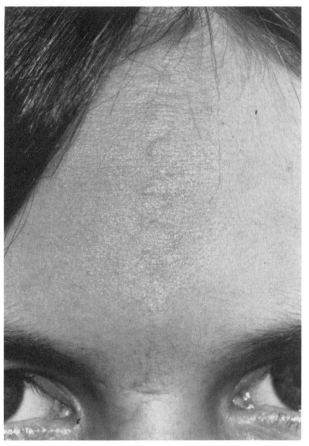

Figure 16b. Post-scar revision, geometric broken line.

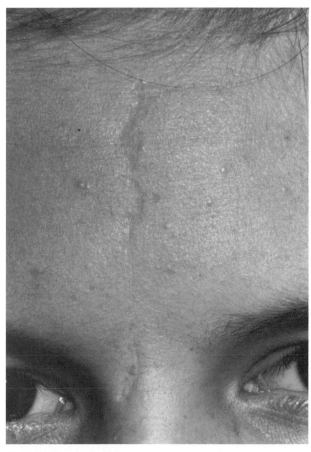

Figure 16a. Forehead scar that is long, wide, depressed, and counter to relaxed skin tension lines.

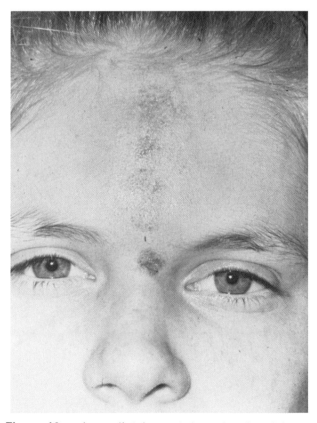

Figure 16c. Immediately post-dermabrasion (photo is overexposed).

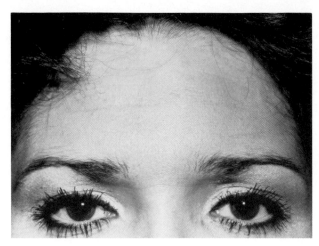

Figure 17b. Post-scar revision (geometric broken line) and dermabrasion.

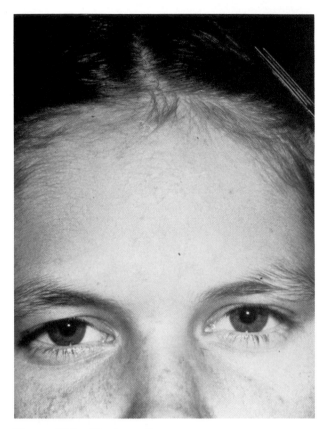

Figure 16d. Final result.

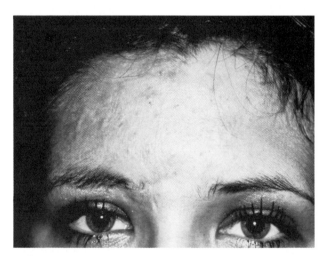

Figure 18a. Forehead windshield glass injury.

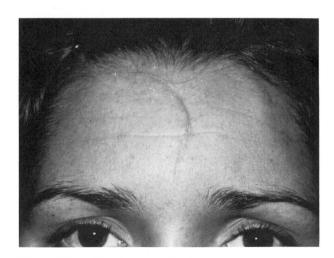

Figure 17a. Forehead vertical scar.

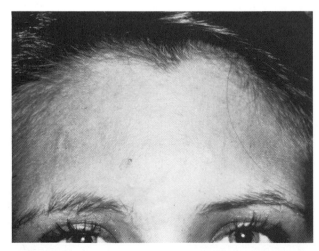

Figure 18b. Post-dermabrasion, no scar revision was required. See text for recommendations for scar revisions.

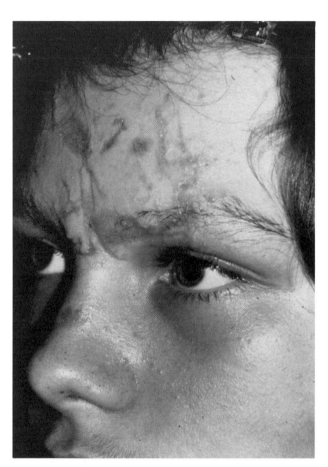

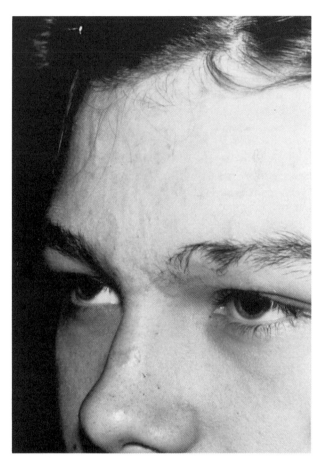

Figure 19a.   Forehead scarring.

Figure 19b.   This patient did not have dermabrasion. This is an example of a case in which time was the best treatment.

When considering a surgical procedure for improvement of a depressed scar, one might first re-excise the scar and approximate the skin edges; then one can dermabrade later, if necessary. In situations where excision is impractical to revise a scar, such as with small depressed acne scars, dermabrasion alone of the scar and the surrounding epidermis might suffice. It is advisable to dermabrade the periphery of the scar to blend with the surrounding tissues.

When treating a circular depressed (ice pick) scar, one could use a punch graft from the post-auricular region to improve the depression first; then the area can be dermabraded three to six months later (Fig. 20).

Grafts can be harvested from the posterior surface of the ear lobules. The donor grafts usually range from the same size to 0.25 or 0.5 mm larger than the recipient site. After graft placement, micropore tape can secure it in position for one week. After one week, the grafts appear dark and crusty. At three weeks, they are pink. Healing is usually complete within three months. Some of the elevation of the grafts is due to edema, which will subside, allowing the graft to flatten over the ensuing three to six months (Fig. 21). For better results, dermaplaning and dermabrasion are usually necessary second and third stages in the patient's treatment program.

TATTOOS

Dermabrasion may also be useful in the removal of tattoos. The more superficially placed tattoos are generally more responsive to dermabrasion due to the fact that most of the pigment is in the superficial layers of the skin. Great care should be taken to leave an ade-

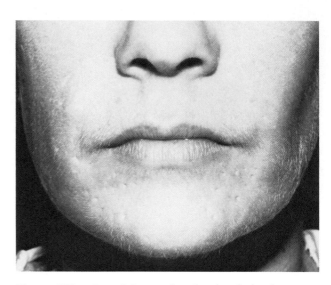

Figure 20b. Ice pick scarring (perioral view).

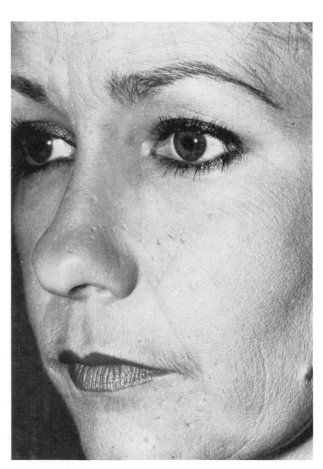

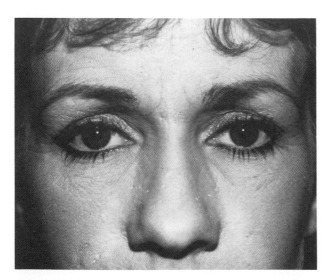

Figure 20a. Ice pick scarring (periorbital and nasal view).

Figure 20c. Ice pick scarring (close-up left oblique view).

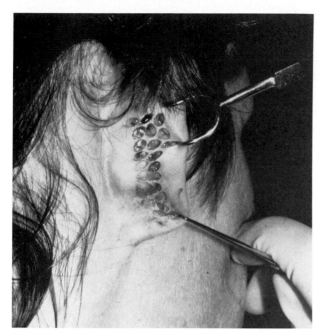

Figure 21a. Donor grafts may be harvested from the post-auricular tissue.

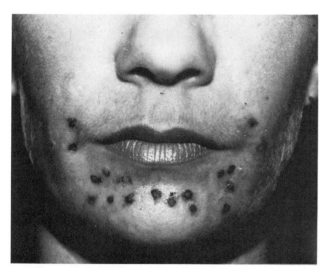

Figure 21b. After one week, the grafts appear dark and crusty.

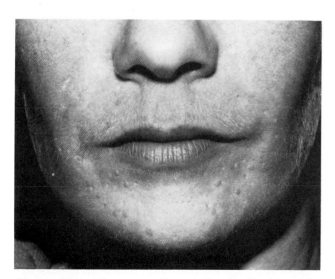

Figure 21c. Three months post-operatively, grafts are well healed, and erythema has faded to a degree.

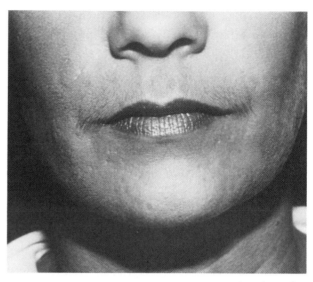

Figure 21d. Two months post-dermabrasion for punch grafts (perioral view).

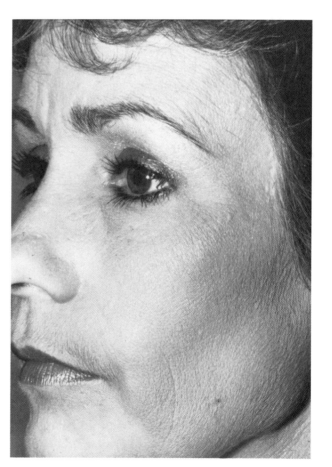

Figure 21e. Two months post-dermabrasion for punch grafts (left oblique view).

21

quate amount of dermal appendages for regeneration. The more professionally placed tattoo pigments are located in the deeper dermis, and are more difficult to remove. If one dermabrades deeply enough to remove all of the pigment, one is likely to remove the dermal appendages and cause scar formation. Another consideration in removing tattoos is the length of time that the tattoo has been present. If even an amateur tattoo has been present for a few months, the pigment may have migrated to a deeper level than originally placed. A deep dermabrasion procedure would be required if total tattoo removal were contemplated.

Consideration should also be given to the location of the tattoo. Generally, tattoos are located in areas other than the face. Most of the face contains relatively thick skin, and is amenable to dermabrasion. On the other hand, if one contemplates treatment of a tattoo located on the inner arm, one must be aware of the increased risk of scar formation, because the skin is so thin and lacks the dermal appendages found in the face. With deep tattoos, the use of a skin graft or serial excision could be considered. If deep dermabrasion is required to remove a tattoo, in many cases, the scarring that could occur might be more or less equivalent to the results obtained with a split-thickness skin graft. However, one could always excise the superficial layers of the scar and place a skin graft over the scar bed.

Dermabrasion is also an excellent method for the treatment of some traumatic tattoos. This can be done either at the time of the initial injury or after healing has occurred. It is more likely to remove the pigment elements if they are treated before the skin has entrapped the pigment. After healing, these pigments can be located as deep, or deeper, than the professionally placed tattoos. The post-dermabrasion regrowth of epidermis from the dermal appendages aids in the camouflage of some of the tattoo material; it may provide enough improvement that total removal is not necessary.

LENTIGENES

Freckles or localized areas of hyperpigmentation can be successfully treated with dermabrasion. Some of the improvement may not be permanent, especially if the excessive pigmentation is located deeply, as with some congenital nevi. With lentigenous lesions, dermabrasion may be as effective as a chemical peel, in that the superficial layer of skin containing the pigment is removed. The permanent removal of the pigmented material is directly related to the depth of the pigment in the skin, and the depth of the surgical insult required in order to remove it (Fig. 22). Deep dermabrasion can be used in lieu of surgical excision for some congenital nevi in children. If necessary,

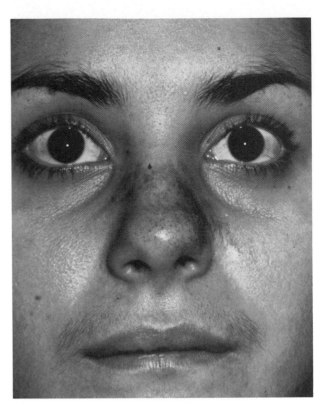

Figure 22a. Congenital nevis (close-up antero-posterior view).

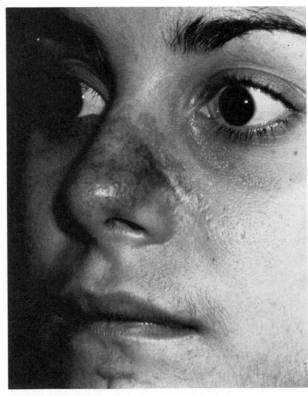

Figure 22b. Congenital nevis (close-up left oblique view).

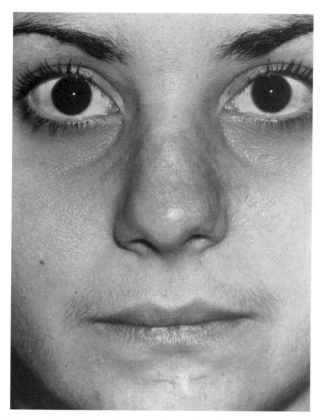

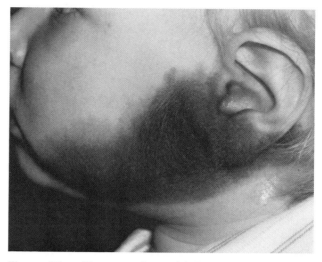

Figure 23a. Young patient with large hairy nevus of the left cheek, mandibular margin region, and ear (April 1981). This case represents an example requiring a combination of techniques (serial excision, skin grafting, dermabrasion).

Figure 22c. Result post-dermabrasion (antero-posterior view).

additional surgery at a later date can be performed (Fig. 23).

FACIAL RHYTIDS

Dermabrasion is occasionally used in treating facial rhytids, especially those located in the forehead, crow's feet of the lateral orbital area, perioral area, and cheeks. Deep horizontal and vertical scar-like wrinkles located in the forehead and nasal labial sulcus cannot be totally removed with this procedure.

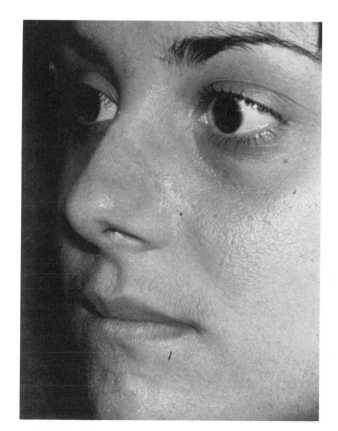

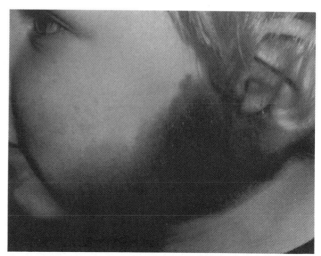

Figure 22d. Result post-dermabrasion (left oblique view).

Figure 23b. Nine months later and pre-operative serial excision (January 1982).

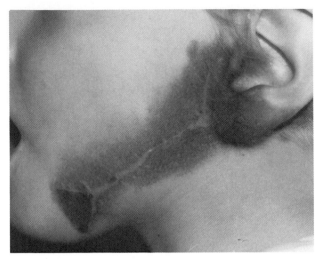

Figure 23c. Five weeks post-operatively, stage 1 serial excision (August 1982).

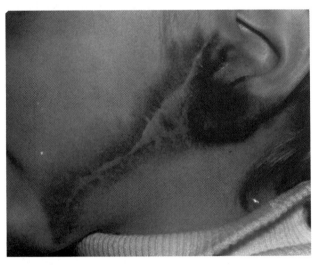

Figure 23d. Four months post-operatively, stage 2 serial excision and full-thickness skin graft to posterior ear (January 1983).

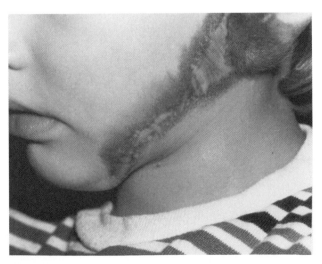

Figure 23e. Eleven months post-operatively, stage 3 serial excision and dermabrasion (September 1984).

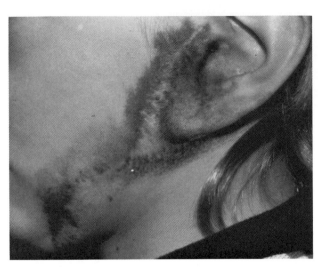

Figure 23f. One year post-operatively, stage 4 dermabrasion (September 1985).

KERATOSES

Seborrheic and actinic keratoses generally respond well to both dermabrasion and chemical peel. Both procedures may decrease the recurrence of keratoses, as well as improve the quality and texture of the skin, resulting in an improved cosmetic and functional result (Figs. 24, 25).

Neither dermabrasion nor chemical peel is generally recommended in the skin of the neck, except in cases where scarring might be anticipated any way (i.e., serial excision or skin grafting). This type of

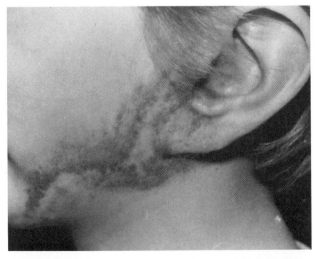

Figure 23g. Post-operatively, stage 5 dermabrasion (September 1986). Patient will require further treatment. Hopefully, the development of the tissue expander will improve the treatment of this type of condition.

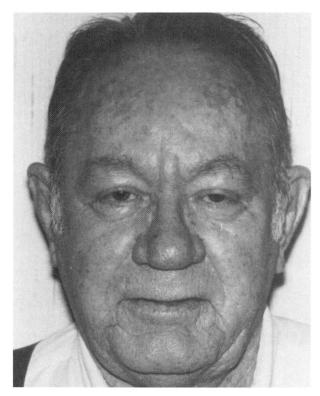

Figure 24a. Patient with actinic keratosis (antero-posterior view).

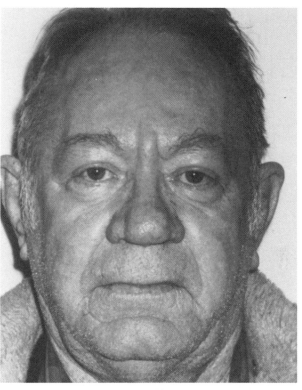

Figure 24c. Post-dermabrasion forehead, with post-chemical peel of the remainder of the face. Moderate improvement of keratosis in this very thick-skinned patient (antero-posterior view).

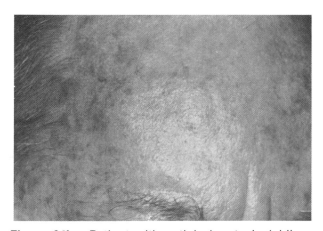

Figure 24b. Patient with actinic keratosis (oblique forehead view).

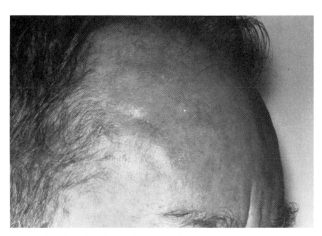

Figure 24d. Oblique forehead view.

insult to the thinner skin of the neck could result in the development of hypertrophic scar formation. The transition between the thinner neck skin and the thicker skin of the face generally occurs at the mandibular margin.

Finally, one must be cautious in patient selection to avoid the emotionally unstable patient and those with unrealistic expectations.

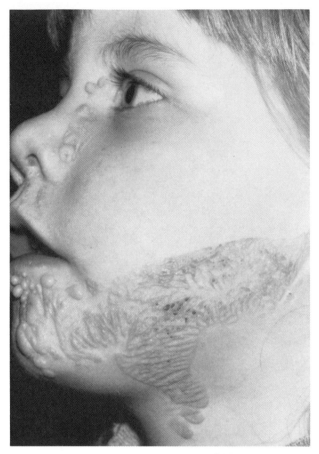

Figure 25b.   Pre-operative view 1-1980.

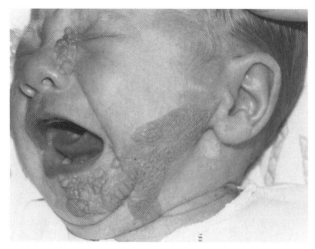

Figure 25a.   Infant with clinical diagnosis of Nevus sebaceous of Jadassohn's; biopsy diagnosis of benign seborrheic keratosis.

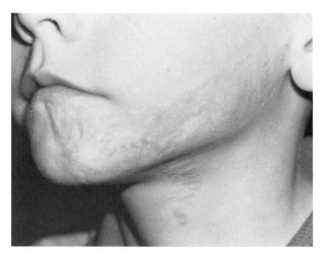

Figure 25c.   Post-operatively staged serial excisions and dermabrasions.

2   Pre-Operative Considerations

The following is our protocol for patients undergoing dermabrasion procedures.

Before surgery, the patient comes to the clinic for a pre-operative evaluation and consultation. Photographs are taken of the face, including anterior-posterior and oblique views, as well as close-ups of selected regions (perioral, periorbital, cheeks, etc.). The patient is given printed material that describes dermabrasion, and is asked to study it and to write down any questions before the consultation. This material assists in preparing the patient for surgery by informing him or her of the limitations of surgery, risks, complications, and alternative methods of treatment. The post-operative instructions and precautions, as well as the possible need for repeated surgery, are reviewed during the consultation. The patient should have a realistic expectation of what dermabrasion might accomplish. The authors try to make the patient understand that perfection can never be achieved. The goal is improvement.

If it is mutually agreed upon between the patient and physician that a dermabrasion procedure is to be performed, patients generally receive prescriptions for a nonaspirin-containing analgesic, multivitamins with a low content of vitamin E, diazepam as a sedative, and tetracycline for prophylactic antibiotic coverage. The patient should begin taking the antibiotic one day before surgery.

When the patient arrives at the clinic on the day of surgery, he or she is given pre-operative medications about one hour before surgery. If the patient is having greater than one third of the face dermabraded, a full pre-operative menu might be given. This generally includes oral dosages of 200 mg Dramamine® (diphenhydramine), 20 mg Valium® (diazepam), and 40 mg prednisone.

The patient washes the face with pHisoderm® before the administration of pre-operative medications. If one third of the face or less is to be dermabraded, the patient is given a smaller amount of pre-operative medication. Only enough oral diazepam is given to sedate the patient for the local anesthetic injections.

After the patient has washed the face and taken pre-operative medications, he or she is moved to the operating suite, and an intravenous line is usually im-

planted. First, 0.10 mg (0.25 cc) scopolamine is given if "twilight sleep" is planned. A cardiac monitor is generally connected to the patient, and then the procedure is begun. The Dermajet containing 2% lidocaine is used to anesthetize the areas of the skin in which regional nerve blocks will be performed.

The entire face is often anesthetized with 1% or 0.5% lidocaine containing 1:100,000 or 1:200,000 epinephrine. Regional blocks may be accomplished on the supraorbital, infraorbital, and mental nerves, if a full-face dermabrasion procedure is to be performed (Fig. 26). From these points, the anesthetic is carried into the other areas that are to be dermabraded (Fig. 27).

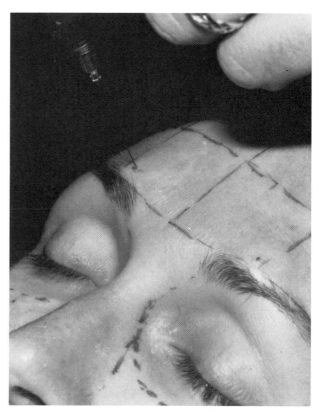

Figure 26a. Supraorbital regional block (regional blocks may help improve patient comfort when large areas are to be anesthetised). (Photo courtesy of Dr. Daniel Russo.)

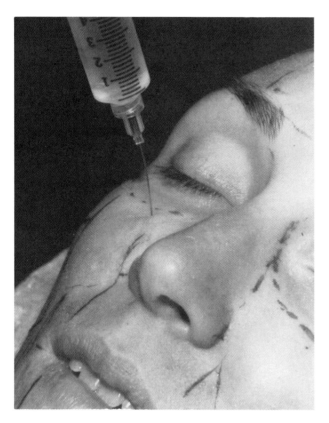

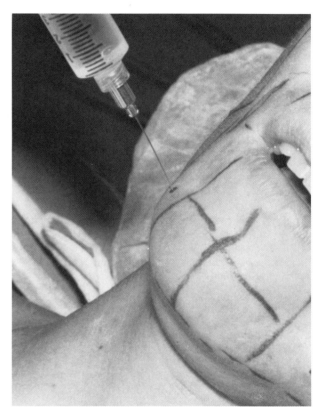

Figure 26b.   Infraorbital regional block. (Photo courtesy of Dr. Daniel Russo.)

Figure 26c.   Mental nerve block. (Photo courtesy of Dr. Daniel Russo.)

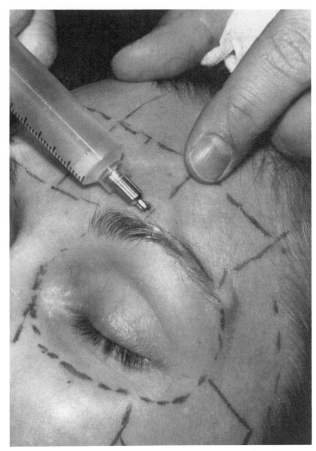

Figure 27a. Anesthetic infiltration is carried from the regional blocks peripherally. (Photo courtesy of Dr. Daniel Russo.)

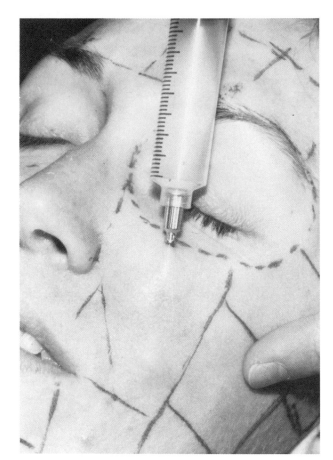

Figure 27b. Close-up view. (Photo courtesy of Dr. Daniel Russo.)

Intravenous diazepam is titrated in 2.5-mg increments to assist in the administration of the local anesthetic injections. The authors generally limit intravenous diazepam to a total of 20 mg. If additional relaxation is required, 0.5 mg hydromorphone may be used. Waiting for at least ten minutes after the administration of the anesthesia allows for the maximum anesthetic effect.

3   Surgical Procedure

Both the surgeon and the surgical assistant should wear eyeglasses or a plastic visor to cover and protect the face and eyes from flying debris removed during the surgical process. One must be constantly aware of the possible transmission of bloodborne disease (such as hepatitis or acquired immune deficiency syndrome [AIDS]) via contact with skin fragments from an affected patient on the conjunctiva of the eye of both the surgeon and/or assistant. A gown should be worn to protect the arms or clothes. Surgical gloves are *advisable,* particularly if the surgeon or assistant has open cuts or abrasions on the hands (Fig. 28).

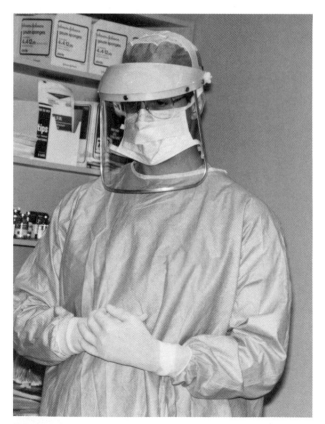

Figure 28. A visor or eyeglasses, surgical gown, gloves, and mask may be advisable due to the possibility of bloodborne diseases.

"Spot" dermabrasion is rarely performed as an initial procedure. The authors generally treat an entire aesthetic facial unit. The color differential of the treated and nontreated areas are more easily camouflaged if facial units, rather than isolated spots, are dermabraded. Some surgeons prefer to dermabrade an entire face to prevent significant pigmentary or texture differentials. In the authors' experience, this is rarely necessary. It may be necessary to dermabrade more deeply in the area of concern, and feather lightly into the area just surrounding the dermabraded area to prevent a significant change in texture or color. If the entire face is treated, it is generally wise to dermabrade more deeply in the areas of focus, and to lightly dermabrade or peel the remainder of the face. In some instances, however, it is impractical to dermabrade the entire face. Small traumatic scars or small isolated acne scars can be dermabraded without much concern. Regardless, the patient should be informed pre-operatively of the possibility of texture and pigmentary changes.

The area to be dermabraded is marked in a grid pattern of 4-cm squares, especially when freezing is used. It has been the authors' experience that if larger areas are frozen, some of the area will have thawed before the dermabrasion can be completed (Fig. 29). Refreezing could result in a deeper surgical insult than desired, increasing the possibility of third-degree injury and scarring. Therefore, we try and limit the freeze to the 4-cm square, so that any refreezing that is done is intentional and not due to excess peripheral freeze.

When treating the full face or cheeks, dermabrasion is usually begun in those squares located in the pre-auricular and mandibular regions. The procedure is gradually continued superiorly and anteriorly. By following this pattern, one can avoid the nuisance of blood running down over the field that is to be abraded next.

After treatment of both cheeks, the chin, and the perioral area, the forehead region is treated. If the nose is to be included in the procedure, it is generally treated last. Often, a periorbital, perioral, and nasal chemical peel may be done before dermabrading to aid in blending when a full-face treatment is consid-

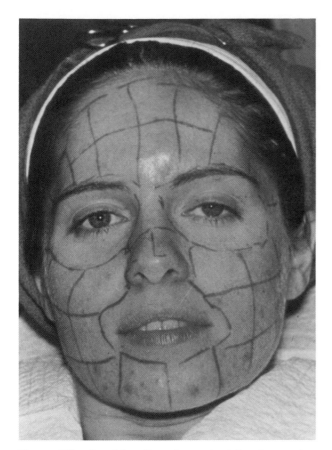

Figure 29. A grid pattern is marked to plan a step-wise dermabrasion. The authors generally try to limit the grid size to 4 cm. Thawing may occur before treatment is completed if larger-size areas are frozen.

ered (Fig. 30). On rare occasions, dermabrasion can be moved into areas that have been peeled, especially in the deeper wrinkles of the forehead and glabella.

Changes in skin texture must be constantly monitored during the dermabrasion procedure to obtain an

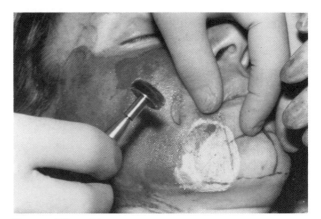

Figure 30b. After treatment of one cheek is completed, the process may be continued around the chin toward the opposite cheek. (Photo courtesy of Dr. Daniel Russo.)

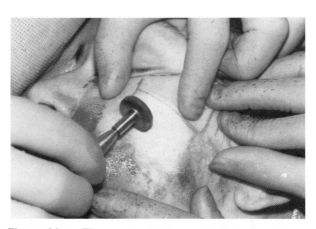

Figure 30c. The pre-auricular and inferiormost segments are treated before the more superior areas to prevent blood from obscuring the surgical field. (Photo courtesy of Dr. Daniel Russo.)

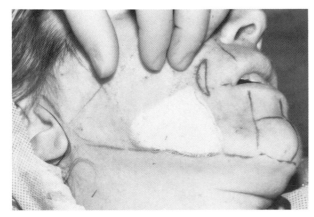

Figure 30a. Treatment is begun in the inferiormost segment of the cheek or pre-auricular region. (Photo courtesy of Dr. Daniel Russo.)

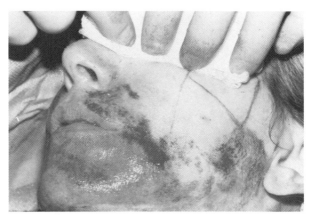

Figure 30d. The treatment is marched superiorly, so that the treatment is performed superior to areas that may be oozing blood. (Photo courtesy of Dr. Daniel Russo.)

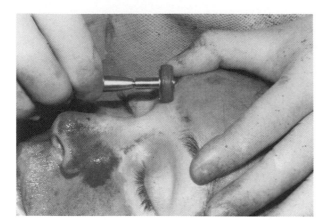

Figure 30e. The forehead is generally treated after both cheeks. This again avoids the nuisance of blood draining over the treatment area. Always ensure that the brush is rotating toward the eyebrows when abrading near this structure. (Photo courtesy of Dr. Daniel Russo.)

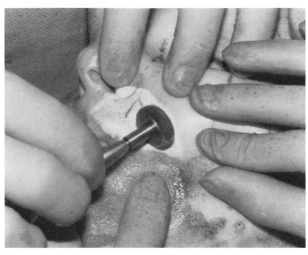

Figure 31. Traction is supplied by the surgeon and assistant. Both must keep their eyes focused on the area being treated to avoid inadvertent injury to the treatment area, surrounding structures, or the operators. All sponges should be removed from the field. A wire brush will "grab" a sponge and could easily cause injury to surgeon, assistant, or patient. (Photo courtesy of Dr. Daniel Russo.)

adequate but safe depth. Both the surgeon and the assistant must always keep their eyes focused on both the dermabrader and the skin to avoid dermabrading too deeply. One must also be cognizant of the fact that adjacent facial structures (eyelids, alae, and lips) could become entwined in the brush or fraise, and be injured or even avulsed (Fig. 31).

When freezing, a barrier should be placed around the periphery of the grid unit to be dermabraded to protect surrounding structures from unnecessary freezing (Fig. 32a). Two freon cans can be used concurrently, especially if a hard freeze is required. This is often the case with the wire brush. The cans are held approximately 2 to 3 inches away from the face; while spraying, they are constantly moved around the grid to be dermabraded in a circular fashion. No ten-

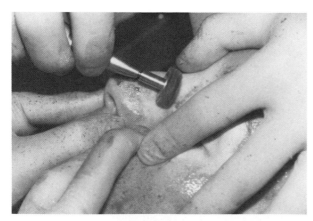

Figure 30f. Adequate stabilization of the nose (traction, support, and freezing) is needed; otherwise, its pliability may allow the brush to pull or tear this structure. (Photo courtesy of Dr. Daniel Russo.)

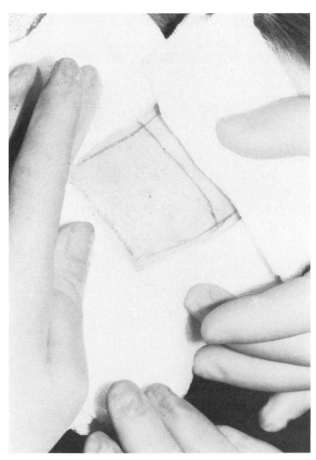

Figure 32a. Sponges are placed around the 4cm grid, when freezing, to protect surrounding structures. All sponges should be removed from the field before dermabrading. (Photo courtesy of Dr. Daniel Russo.)

sion or countertraction is applied to the surrounding skin during freezing, so that the skin is allowed to freeze in its normal anatomic position. After the skin becomes completely white, as a result of the formation of ice crystals, the surgeon is advised to gently tap the surface of the skin (Figs. 32b, c). If no indentation is made as one taps with the finger, then freezing is adequate. At this time, *all* sponges are removed from the area to be dermabraded; otherwise, the wire brush could quickly grab any gauze that is near the field, thereby causing the dermabrader to run across the face and injure the patient or damage the dermabrading instrument. After all gauze sponges are removed, the surgeon and assistant turn their attention to the area surrounding the surgical grid unit.

The dermabrasion unit should be held firmly between the fingers, especially when using the wire brush. The wire brush has a tendency to travel off course if the unit is not firmly gripped. Should this unfortunate event occur, one could produce a deep groove or scar in the patient's skin (Fig. 33).

The unit should be held in a position so that the wheel is perpendicular to the plane of the patient's

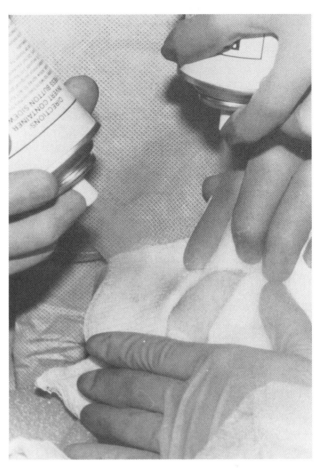

Figure 32c. We usually have both the surgeon and the assistant spray the frigiderm. This helps shorten the freezing interval, providing more efficient use of operating time.

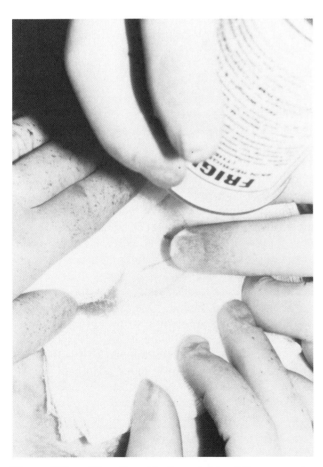

Figure 32b. After the skin becomes white, one may gently tap the skin to determine the firmness. If one tests the skin too soon, an indentation may freeze into place. (Photo courtesy of Dr. Daniel Russo.)

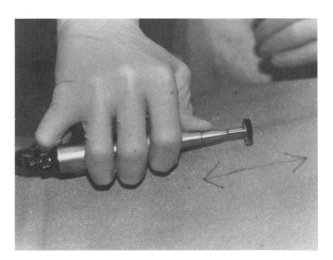

Figure 33. A firm grip is essential for the safe use of the instrument. The use of the wire brush should encourage added precautions. It has a tendency to grab and pull. The authors tend to abrade in a direction perpendicular (medial and lateral) to the rotation of the brush (see arrows). The diamond fraise may also "grab" gauze.

skin. While the skin is being stabilized with countertraction administered by the assistant, the surgeon should be protecting the eyes, nose, and mouth with his or her hand. Gauze should never be used to protect these areas due to the potential danger of snaring with the wire brush (Fig. 34).

The authors use a wire brush for most dermabrasions. The brush generally achieves the required depth more quickly than the diamond fraise, and creates multiple incisions into the dermis that release scar contractures, thereby allowing the new epidermis to bridge the spaces. This phenomenon results in a smoother skin texture when healing is complete. The diamond fraise planes the skin more slowly, but has the advantage of not requiring the hard freeze that is sometimes needed with the wire brush.

The diamond fraise is sometimes used when dermabrading small, hard-to-reach areas, such as the groove of the nasal alae. It is also employed in the rare situation where dermabrasion is required near the eyelids (Fig. 35).

By using the diamond fraise, the inexperienced surgeon may find it easier to follow the depth of tissue insult as the dermabrasion procedure progresses.

Initially, one observes removal of the epidermal layer containing the surface pigment. As dermabrasion is continued, the small blood vessels disappear, and one can visualize the appearance of small openings in the sebaceous glands. Still deeper, small yellow patches of the sebaceous glands become more apparent. When these landmarks are recognizable, the plane of abrasion is still within the upper layers of

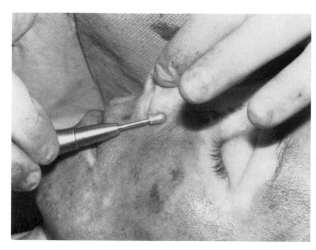

Figure 35. The small pear-shaped diamond fraise is used for hard to reach areas, such as the groove around the nasal alae. (Photo courtesy of Dr. Daniel Russo.)

the dermis. When the yellow patches disappear, one has reached the lower dermis. Dermabrading beyond this area increases the risk for post-operative hypertrophic scar formation. If the procedure were to continue, one would quickly encounter the subcutaneous fat. It is therefore advisable to limit the dermabrasion procedure to the superficial and mid-dermis. Since the diamond fraise allows one to follow the layers more clearly, it is generally safe for use by an inexperienced surgeon. Even though the procedure progresses more slowly, this added safety factor may prevent disaster, especially until one has obtained experience in performing this procedure.

When using a wire brush for dermabrasion, it is also possible to follow the layers in the stepwise manner described previously.

Caution should be observed when dermabrading in the groove between the lip and the chin and over the nose. These areas are difficult to stabilize with countertraction. If the skin is not held taut, one increases the risk of the brush or fraise digging too deeply into the skin in these regions. Another area for concern is in the mandibular region. This area and others over bony prominences are naturally more prone to excessive scar formation following injury. This phenomenon may be due to the fact that the skin is thin, and that this skin is constantly under additional tension with movements of the head and neck. Skin overlying bone tends to freeze more rapidly; therefore, some of the tissue insult may be due to excessive freezing. When the surgeon dermabrades around any orifice (lips or eyes), one must position the dermabrasion unit so that the cutting part of the wheel is rotating toward the orifice. This practice tends to prevent the brush from grabbing and retracting the lip or eyelid away from the orifice. In this situation, it would be

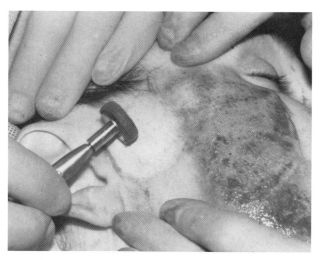

Figure 34. The brush is held perpendicular to the skin. It is moved in a back-and-forth direction (see Fig. 33). Abrasion is begun around the periphery of the frozen grid and worked toward the center (the center is usually the last to thaw). Note that the brush is held so that it rotates toward the hair of the sideburn to prevent entanglement. (Photo courtesy of Dr. Daniel Russo.)

easy to tear the skin, and/or avulse an eyelid or lip (Figs. 36a, b, c).

When using a wire brush, it is generally helpful to freeze the skin until it is firm, because the brush has a tendency to drag and dig into the tissues. The procedure is begun at the periphery of each frozen grid unit, and progresses toward the center, which is usually the last area to thaw. The unit is firmly held between the fingers, and should be swept in a back-and-forth horizontal fashion (Fig. 33). One develops a "feel" for brushing away the superficial or irregular layers of the skin, as if one were sanding a rough surface of a piece of wood furniture, removing scratches and dents. One can also use small circular motions over skin that is firmly stabilized.

If one dermabrades in a single direction, it is possible to leave behind ridges or high spots. These could be smoothed by either dermabrading gently over the ridges or turning the unit so that dermabrasion is performed lightly at right angles to the original direction.

For the inexperienced surgeon, it is essential that he or she practices before performing a first dermabrasion procedure on a patient. Grapefruit can be used to learn the proper method for holding the unit, and to improve one's technical skills. This laboratory model will provide much of the feeling obtained by dermabrading human skin. It is wise to observe as many procedures as possible that are performed by an expert in dermabrasion, either via videotape or in per-

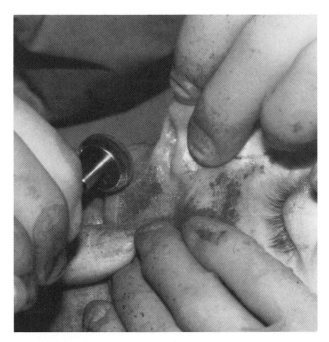

Figure 36b.   The brush is rotating (abrading) toward the lip. (Photo courtesy of Dr. Daniel Russo.)

son. By observing many procedures and practicing on a grapefruit, the surgeon can be better prepared to perform this procedure for the first time on a patient. This can also help one to recognize when an adequate depth has been reached.

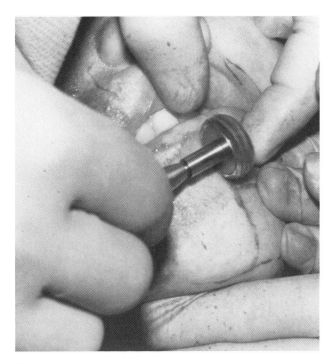

Figure 36a.   The area between the lip and chin is difficult to stabilize. The skin should be held as taut as possible to help prevent abrading too deeply. Note that the brush is rotating toward the lip. (Photo courtesy of Dr. Daniel Russo.)

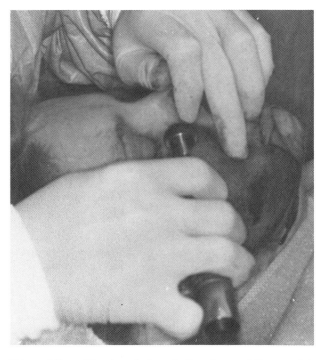

Figure 36c.   The brush is rotating toward the eyelid when treating the infraorbital region. The thin structures can easily be snagged and torn. Note, the surgeon does not abrade the eyelid with the wire brush.

At the conclusion of the procedure, the authors generally apply wet saline gauze over the treated areas to absorb the initial oozing of blood and serum (Figs. 37a, b). If the patient is free of clotting abnormalities, there should be no problem with continuous bleeding after ten minutes have passed. The authors prefer to observe the patient for 60 to 90 minutes after the procedure. The intravenous line is then removed. In the authors' practice, the patient generally remains at or near the clinic overnight when large areas have been dermabraded and a full anesthetic menu has been given. In such cases, the patient is examined the following morning. Many surgeons, however, allow patients to go home, when stable, following the procedure.

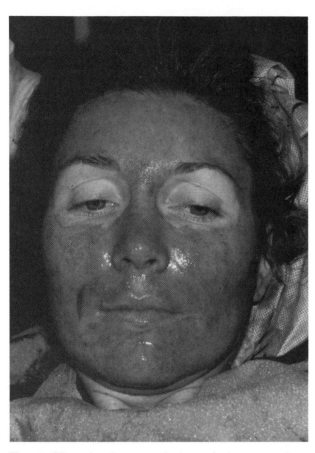

Figure 37a. At the completion of the procedure, there will be some oozing of blood and serum. (Photo courtesy of Dr. Daniel Russo.)

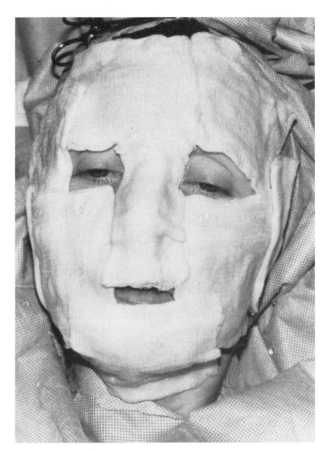

Figure 37b. Wet saline gauze sponges are used to absorb any drainage and to keep the wounds moist. These are changed hourly the night after surgery. (Photo courtesy of Dr. Daniel Russo.)

4 Post-Operative Considerations

After surgery, the patient uses moistened gauze sponges on the treated areas. These moist sponges (Fig. 37b) are replaced hourly to prevent adherence to the abraded regions. If the patient goes home, or a family member stays with the patient to change the gauze pads, they should understand that the sponges tend to stick to the treated areas if left on too long. If it should occur, however, the gauze can be gently teased away if remoistened. Both the patient and family should also know that during the first 24 hours, the dermabraded areas may ooze a yellow serum. They should not become alarmed about this normal part of the healing process.

The morning following surgery, patients should begin daily washings consisting of six evenly spaced showers with body temperature tap water. After each shower, the patient applies a thin layer of a vitamin A- and E-enriched vegetable oil-type cream (Dermed®), or with Crisco® shortening. Both moisturize the skin surface and help prevent drying and crusting (Fig. 38). This routine is continued for the first 7 to 14 days, or until the initial healing is complete; then the patient may begin to wear makeup. Water-based makeups are recommended early on. They can be easily removed with water (Fig. 39).

Patients should be informed that the skin will be deep pink or red in color for the first two weeks, but that this will gradually fade. For several months post-operatively, the skin will demonstrate some red or pink discoloration. This usually subsides, however, after about eight weeks. Patients should understand that they must avoid sunlight for at least two full

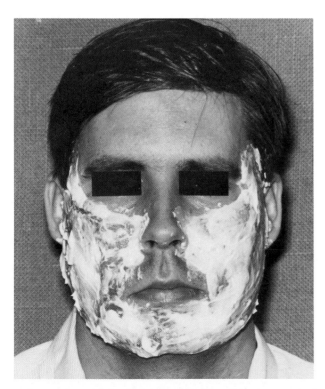

Figure 38a. After each shower, the face is covered with a layer of vegetable oil-type cream. Ensure that the cream is generously applied.

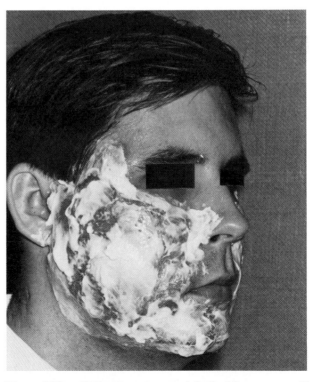

Figure 38b. Patients may complain that the cream will not "stick" or cannot be evenly applied. This is due to the early oozing of tissue serum and will subside.

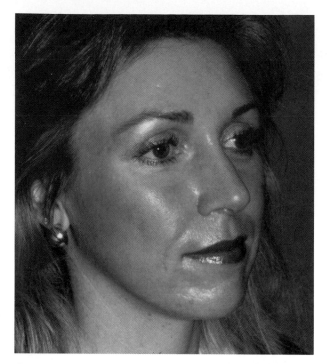

Figure 39. There will be some erythema for several weeks post-dermabrasion. Water-based hypoallergenic makeup may be used (two weeks post-operatively). (Photo courtesy of Dr. Daniel Russo.)

months. After that time, they may protect the skin with a sunscreen containing at least a #15 sun protection factor. Sunscreens should be used outdoors for at least six months post-operatively. It is much safer for the patient to avoid direct sunlight, in addition to using sunscreen for the full six-month period. If they do not follow the above instructions, they should know that hyperpigmentation may occur.

The new skin is very delicate—like that of a newborn baby; therefore, patients may need to use bland hypoallergenic skin moisturizers for a period after surgery. The texture of the *new* skin will be different from the nontreated areas, and makeup may be required to camouflage this. About six months after surgery, the new skin is generally mature enough to toughen and endure graduated exposure to the elements (sun, heat, cold, and wind). Because contact dermatitis is more likely to occur with this new delicate skin, patients must avoid materials containing harsh chemicals for at least six months.

During the first night following the dermabrasion procedure, patients may experience some mild stinging or moderate throbbing in the treated areas. Most patients, however, have *no* discomfort. If a patient does, however, a mild analgesic or saline-cooled compresses may help to relieve any discomfort.

Moderate-to-severe swelling follows, especially if the dermabrasion encircles the eyes or the lips. The edema usually reaches its peak on the second or third day post-operatively, but begins to subside on the fourth or fifth day. Elevation of the head of the bed and staying upright during waking hours will also tend to improve the situation.

The patient should be instructed not to pull off any crust that may develop. This may remove some of the new skin attached to the undersurface of the crusts and delay healing, or even produce scarring. In addition, patients should also be instructed not to wear shower caps or hair pieces over treated areas, because they could produce pressure that could delay healing or produce scarring.

Milia may be seen during the first two months post-operatively. Most of these disappear without treatment. If, however, some remain, they can be easily uncapped with a #18 gauge needle (Fig. 40). The patient should also be informed that any emotional upset or exposure of the face to cold, heat, wind, or sun may cause temporary erythema.

Depression is occasionally seen in post-dermabrasion patients. This is secondary to the traumatic effects of seeing a swollen, discolored face, as well as the residual effects of the operative medications—a "hangover" of sorts.

Erythema is not really a complication. It is an *expected* sequela of both dermabrasion and chemical peel. It is more apparent during the first two weeks post-operatively and gradually subsides. There will usually be a pink color to the skin for about two months after surgery. This phenomenon is accentuated with exposure to the sun, wind, cold, and heat. Excessive freezing during the dermabrasion procedure may accentuate the post-operative erythema. In any event, this condition usually resolves with proper skin protection and care.

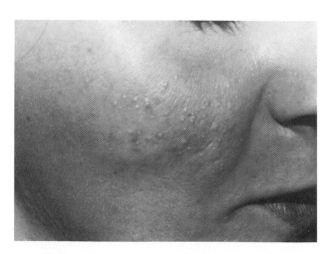

Figure 40. Milia may be easily removed with a #18 gauge needle (see milia in Fig. 41c).

Despite all side effects, the patient is usually ready to return to work within two weeks post-operatively, and generally experiences, with an improvement in the skin texture, an increased self-esteem. Patients should be aware of the lag time for maximum benefits of dermabrasion. They cannot expect an immediate improvement. It often takes several weeks for the new collagen formation to be completed. At this time, the improvement in the quality and texture of the skin can be appreciated, assuming no complications occurred during healing.

To help promote healing, the authors employ the moist-dressing technique described previously; that is, multiple washings and bland creams. With this routine, healing occurs more rapidly. This principle has been well described by Maibach and Rovee.[1] The problem of localized infections is rarely observed using the "open" method.

5 Contraindications

Table 2 lists some relative contraindications to dermabrasion.

DARK- OR OLIVE-COLORED SKIN

Dark- or olive-colored skin is a relative contraindication to dermabrasion due to the high probability of post-operative pigmentary changes in the treated areas. A black patient with acne scarring may benefit from dermabrasion, but he or she must accept the possibility that the color of the treated area may differ from the rest of the face. In cases of severe scarring, any hyperpigmentation that may occur is generally no more disfiguring than the scarring for which the procedure was performed to achieve a better texture (Figs. 41, 42).

Pustular Acne

Localized infections such as pustular acne are first treated medically with facial cleansing solutions and antibiotics before surgery.

SKIN OF THE NECK

Dermabrasion is usually discouraged on the thin skin of the neck. As mentioned earlier, the skin along the mid-portion of the mandible is more susceptible to hypertrophic scarring when the deepest dermal layers are penetrated. The unusual tension placed on this region, with normal movements of the head during the day and while sleeping on the side at night, may be a contributing factor. Caution should always be maintained when planing over bony prominences. In these regions, this skin is often less mobile; therefore, the layers may be cut more quickly with abrading. Deep dermabrasion alone does not necessarily result in hypertrophic scarring. On the other hand, when a deep dermabrasion is needed, one must be cautious not to extend the procedure below the dermis.

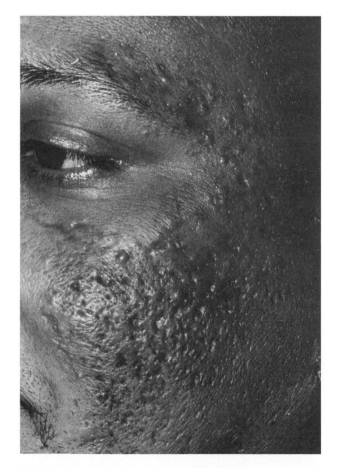

Figure 41a. Pre-operative black patient with severe cystic acne and acne scarring. In this case, the benefits of dermabrasion outweigh any possibility of pigmentary changes.

Table 2. Relative Contraindications for Dermabrasion

Dark or olive-colored skin

Skin of the neck

Pustular acne

Keloids and/or hypertrophic scars

Unrealistic patient expectations

Use of hormone-containing medications (estrogen, progesterone)

Active herpetic lesions (fever blisters)

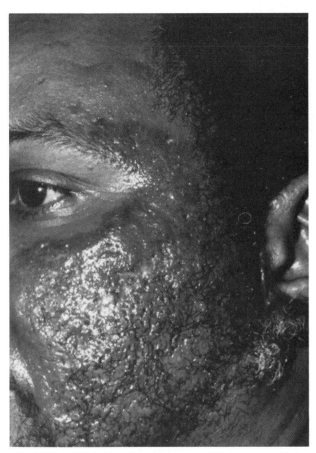

Figure 41b. Hyperpigmentation at one month post-operatively.

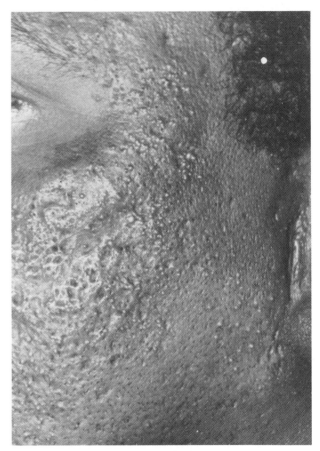

Figure 41c. Significant resolution of hyperpigmentation two months post-operatively. Note milia.

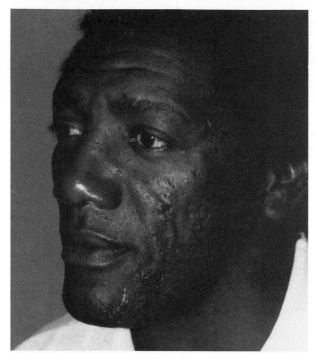

Figure 42a. Black patient with severe cystic acne and acne scarring. Benefits of therapeutic dermabrasion outweigh any possible pigmentary changes. The patient has endured years of troublesome cystic acne. (Photo courtesy of Dr. Daniel Russo.)

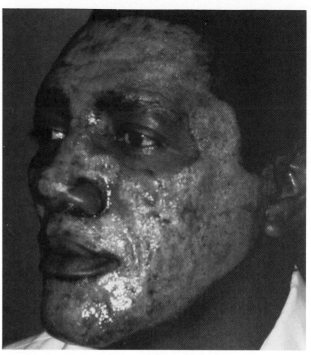

Figure 42c. One day post-operatively. Removal of pigmented skin contrasts sharply with untreated areas. (Photo courtesy of Dr. Daniel Russo.)

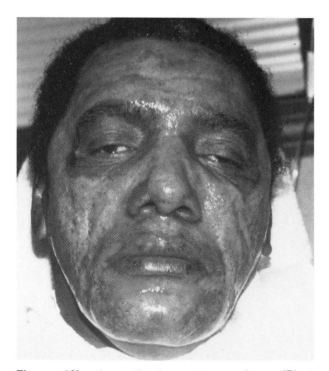

Figure 42b. Immediately post-procedure. (Photo courtesy of Dr. Daniel Russo.)

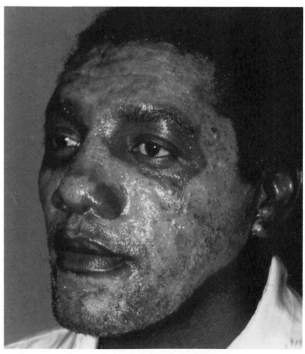

Figure 42d. One week post-operatively. (Photo courtesy of Dr. Daniel Russo.)

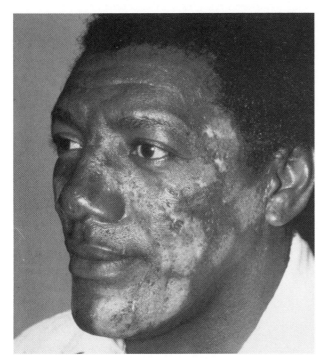

Figure 42e. One month post-operatively. Pigmentation is returning. Note several areas of hypopigmentation. (Photo courtesy of Dr. Daniel Russo.)

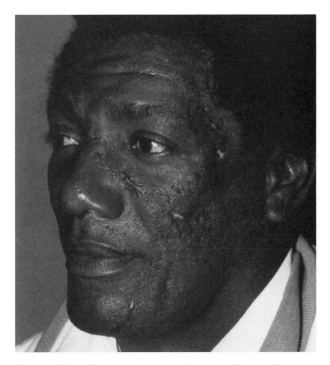

Figure 42f. Three months post-operatively. Pigmentation is returning. Note the improvement of acne along the margin of the mandible. The patient will require further wound maturation and additional treatment. (Photo courtesy of Dr. Daniel Russo.)

KELOIDS AND/OR HYPERTROPHIC SCARS

Hypertrophic scarring is a rare complication. It most often occurs when dermabrasion is performed too deeply or in areas with very thin skin. Post-operative infection and iatrogenic trauma, such as scratching the crusted areas with fingernails or by picking off crusts, can also lead to hypertrophic scarring.

Keloids and/or hypertrophic scars should not be dermabraded. The growth of a keloid may be stimulated. The authors believe that neither of these types of scars are amenable to dermabrasion. Wide scars, deep burns, or skin with congenitally absent or iatrogenically reduced skin appendages (X-ray therapy), represent situations in which dermabrasion is generally contraindicated. It must be noted that skin appendages are necessary for regeneration of the epidermis. In each of the described situations, the appendages are either dminished or absent.

UNREALISTIC PATIENT EXPECTATIONS

A major contraindication is the unrealistic and unreliant patient. Expecting more than the procedure can deliver is common in patients seeking dermabrasion. Regardless of how well the limitations are explained pre-operatively, patients generally expect results that are rarely obtainable. A good physician-patient relationship is critical *prior* to the procedure. Both surgeon and patient should have a clear understanding of the procedure, post-operative care, and post-operative appearance. The patient should also understand that some degree of pigmentary change is expected. In addition, they must be willing to follow the post-operative instructions very closely, and to understand that they must protect themselves from the sun for at least six months post-operatively. The post-operative instructions recommended by the authors for patients who have had dermabrasion are included in Chapter 7.

HORMONE-CONTAINING MEDICATIONS

The use of estrogen- or progesterone-containing medications during the postoperative period may result in pigmentary changes. The authors generally instruct dermabrasion patients to discontinue any estrogen- or progesterone-containing medications or birth control pills for 6 months postoperatively.

HERPETIC LESIONS

The presence of fever blisters is a contraindication to dermabrasion. The vesicles may spread to any area which is treated. If the patient has no visable lesions but has a past history of them, the authors generally use Zovirax® 200 mg poq 4° × 7 days as a prophylactic measure.

6   Complications

In the authors' experience, infection has rarely been seen with the moist-dressing method for post-operative care. If infection should occur, however, it is usually the result of an individual patient not following the directions for cleaning the face.

Insufficient treatment or persistent irregularities should not be considered a complication of dermabrasion. If a surgeon is inexperienced at performing the dermabrasion procedure, it is best to be conservative. If necessary, the surgeon would need to redermabrade the area. Generally, if healing occurs within five days post-therapy, only a superficial layer of skin was removed. A properly performed dermabrasion procedure should require 10 to 14 days for healing to be completed.

Some pigmentary changes usually follow dermabrasion, especially in darker-skinned individuals. Hyperpigmentation can also be seen in fair-skinned individuals who expose themselves to sunlight. This problem, however, can usually be diminished by adequate sun protection (Fig. 43). *Hypopigmentation occurs most often when the dermabrasion and/or freezing is performed at the deeper layers,* thereby destroying melanocytes in the lower levels of the dermis. If the patient has areas of spotty hyperpigmentation at one year post-operatively, this may be improved by the careful and accurate application of a chemical peel solution or by an additional dermabrasion procedure.

If a large area is treated in the initial dermabrasion procedure, it may be wise to dermabrade and/or peel the remainder of the face to achieve greater uniformity in the overall texture and quality of the skin. In many cases, this reduces the possibility of noticeable pigmentary disparities.

Some observers have noted a significant delay in healing in patients who have recently used Accutane® (isotretinoin) for the treatment of acne. This drug appears to decrease sebaceous gland function and delay keratinization. As discussed previously, the pilosebaceous apparatus is required in the skin regeneration process. If Accutane® has been used within the past six months, it is conceivable that there may not be adequate recovery of the activity of epithelial-regenerating components to foster post-operative healing. It may be wise to consult a

dermatologist with regard to dermabrading a patient who has been treated with Accutane.®

Herpetic eruptions may occur especially if the patient has a prior history of fever blisters. If ulcerations develop, oral Zovirax® 200 mg poq 4° may be used along with topical Zovirax® ointment.

Erythema may persist beyond the 3-month period in hypersensitive individuals. Should this occur, time, reassurance, and 2.5% hydrocortisone cream will help.

Scarring may occur if dermabrasion is carried too deeply or if embedded scar tissue secondary to acne or other processes is encountered during the planing process. Some scarring may be unavoidable when treat-

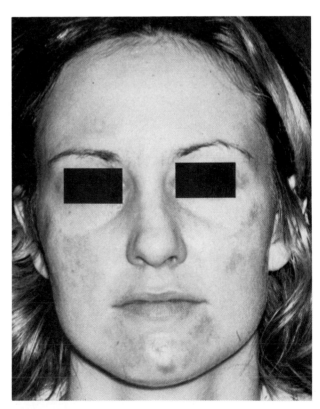

Figure 43. Post-dermabrasion hyperpigmentation. Time and adequate sun protection can usually alleviate this condition.

45

ing severe acne cases. Severe post-op infections or iatrogenic damage secondary to scratching or pulling crusts may also result in scarring.

Milia may occur during the post-operative period. This usually resolves with postoperative cleaning. A #18 gauge needle may be used to uncap persistent cysts.

URTICARIA OR CONTACT DERMATITIS

Urticaria or contact dermatitis may occur in some hypersensitive patients after the dermabrasion procedure (or peel). The etiology of allergic dermatitis is unknown, but may be related to intractable diaper rash in the newborn. Antihistamines and dilute concentrations of nonfluorinated topical steroids may be helpful in this situation. If the physician is not a dermatologist, consultation with one is often necessary.

When contact dermatitis occurs, the following regimen has proven to be effective in helping the patient with supersensitive skin through the initial healing period.

Contact Dermatitis Treatment Regimen

Following chemical peel or dermabrasion, use:

1. 0.25% Acetic acid soak—mix 1 tbsp of white vinegar with 1 pt of water.
2. 1% Hytone cream.
3. Eucerin cream.
4. Delclens soap.

Directions

1. Use acetic acid soak on a clean washcloth for 5 to 15 minutes. Gently place this on the affected area twice per day. Do not rub or wipe the cloth on affected areas.
2. Cover red areas with 1% hytone cream twice per day.
3. Use Eucerin cream to moisturize as needed over the rash. Apply gently with a patting technique.
4. When washing the face, use Delclens soap. Use no more than twice per day.

7 Post-Dermabrasion Instructions: A Guide for the Patient

The following instructions are based on experience with hundreds of dermabrasions and are designed to answer patient questions regarding the "do's" and "don't's" following this procedure. Both the patient and family should read this section several times and become thoroughly familiar with its contents. It has been the authors' experience that *faithful* adherence to these instructions tends to result in the smoothest post-operative course and promote most favorable healing. Whenever a question arises, refer back to this chapter; more than likely, one will find the answer. If one is still unsure, by all means, the patient should telephone the physician.

PAIN

There may be some moderate throbbing and mild stinging following dermabrasion, but most patients feel the procedure is surprisingly pain-free. Discomfort can usually be relieved by taking one or two of the prescribed pain tablets, and by the application of cooled compresses during this time. A convenient way to fashion the compresses is to place crushed ice in a small plastic zip-lock bag, which can be obtained at most grocery stores. The ice compresses should be discontinued after the stinging subsides.

Any additional discomfort should be relieved by an oral pain medication. (If the patient has had any additional procedures, however, he or she should check the instructions for that procedure and make sure it is permissible to take aspirin.) The patient should use one of the *nonaspirin* pain relievers if he or she is unsure (Tylenol®, Anacin-3®, or Percogesic®).

SWELLING

The patient can expect a moderate-to-severe amount of swelling. This will be especially true if the areas around the eyes and lips have been treated. Remember, this is only temporary. It will be the greatest by the second or third day and should begin to subside by the fourth or fifth day.

One can help decrease the amount of swelling by keeping the head elevated about 30 to 40° when lying down and, by staying up (sitting, standing, or walking around) as much as possible for the next three or four days. Sometimes medications may be given to help reduce the swelling.

Some degree of swelling follows any surgical procedure. The swelling is due to the new tissue fluids brought into the area by the body to promote healing. The increased blood supply to the region is responsible for the pink color of the skin and some of the "discoloration" associated with surgery. When these healing fluids are no longer required, the tissues release them and they are absorbed through the bloodstream.

One must be willing to accept temporary swelling and discoloration, which occurs following such procedures. Although usually visually disconcerting, most patients feel it is a negligible inconvenience to pay for the physical and psychological improvement they generally experience.

SKIN APPEARANCE AND CARE

Shortly, after surgery, the patient will notice that the dermabraded area resembles a "skinned knee," and one may notice yellow-colored fluid oozing from the skin. This is part of the normal healing process. However, it usually subsides within 24 hours. *When it subsides,* one should begin gently washing the dermabraded area with body temperature tap water. This is most easily accomplished by standing in a shower and using only the finger tips. Do *not* use a wash cloth or soap. *This washing must be repeated six times per day.*

Following each washing, the prescribed ointment or cream must be applied to the dermabraded areas like a *light* layer of frosting on a cake. This acts as a moisturizer and is designed to prevent dryness and crusting.

Never pick at crusts that do not loosen easily. Apply 47

the prescribed cream to them liberally, and they should come off with time. (Avoid getting creams or ointment in the eyes.) At this time in the healing process, new delicate skin is being formed, and premature removal of the crusts may damage this tender new skin and delay healing.

Do not wear a shower cap or hair piece that contacts any area that has been dermabraded, as this might result in delayed healing and jeopardize an otherwise good result.

By about the 10th to 14th day, most of the crusting should have disappeared. The new skin will appear intensely pink. At this stage, the moistening agent should be applied more sparingly, but be gently rubbed in, much in the manner one would use a moisturizing cream.

Within about 14 days, the patient should be able to use makeup over the dermabraded areas, but one should not do this alone. It will be discussed during follow-up visits, and specific recommendations will be made at that time. Although they do not usually cover as well, water-based makeups are more easily removed, and are therefore recommended for the first week or so that makeup is used. Makeup is never applied to unhealed areas or crusts.

The intense pink color usually fades after the second week, but some pink will remain for about six to eight weeks. After the pink color disappears, the skin usually remains more tense and somewhat smoother.

Occasionally, small "white cysts" may appear in the treated areas. These usually disappear in two or three weeks without specific treatment. If they do not, the physician can show the patient how to eradicate them.

Early in the healing process, exposure to heat, cold, wind, or emotional upset (fear, anger, crying, etc.) will cause the skin to temporarily become intensely pink. This is due to increased blood flow or "blushing." After about three or four months, this phenomenon should disappear.

FEVER BLISTERS

Patients who have *ever* had difficulty with "fever blisters" or "cold sores" may develop an exacerbation of these lesions four or five days after surgery. If one has ever had this problem, one should take Zovirax®, one tablet six times per day for the first week post-operatively. This can be prescribed by your physician. You will be given a one-week supply. Should blisters definitely appear, the patient should call the physician so that medications may be prescribed to be applied to the affected areas four times per day. The authors feel this may help prevent spreading of the "fever blisters" and often relieves some of the discomfort. The authors are not aware of any permanent effects of these fever blisters when these instructions have been followed.

MEDICATIONS

When the patient is released following surgery, he or she should continue taking medicines prescribed prior to the dermabrasion—take them as directed until the supply is exhausted; these prescriptions do not need to be refilled. One may also be given several new prescriptions at the time of discharge. One of them is for the relief of any discomfort being experienced. This has been discussed in the section on "Pain." A sleeping pill may also be prescribed and should not be filled unless the patient feels they are needed.

Sometimes an antibiotic will be given. If these are prescribed, they should be started immediately and should be taken until the supply is finished. If one has a history of "fever blister" or "cold sores," other medications may be prescribed as mentioned in the section on "Fever Blisters."

DEPRESSION

Because a person is so "keyed-up" before surgery, there is usually a mental and physical let-down afterward. It is not unusual for the patient to feel depressed and tired following surgery. If this happens, do not be concerned.

No matter how much they wanted the procedure beforehand and how much they were informed about what to expect post-operatively, most patients are still surprised when they see their face swollen and discolored. One usually looks worse for a few days following dermabrasion. The patient needs to realize that every other patient experiences the same feelings. The best "treatment" is to busy one's self with post-operative care and diverting one's attention to other activities (TV, books, etc.).

RESUMING ACTIVITIES

Wearing Eyeglasses

If the nose area has been dermabraded, one should wait two weeks before wearing eyeglasses. The pressure of glasses resting on the dermabraded nose skin (except for very brief periods of time) is to be avoided.

Sun Exposure

Try to avoid direct and indirect rays of the sun for at least eight weeks. Blotchy pigmentation of the dermabraded areas may appear if the new delicate skin is exposed too early. This means that exposure to the sun (golfing, fishing, tennis, similar activities) during the sunny part of the day should be avoided during the initial eight-week period. The dermabraded areas should be protected for six months by large-brimmed hats and a sun screen product (such as Sundown®, Supershade®, or a similar product) if one is to be exposed for prolonged periods—use the most potent concentration in the beginning.

Skin Care

Continued use of skin moisturizers will be the best adjunct in nurturing the new skin and preserving its smooth and soft texture.

Returning to Work and Resuming Social Activities

When those should commence depends upon the amount of public contact and amount of sun exposure one's job involves, plus the degree of redness and swelling that develops. The average patient returns to work or goes out socially about two weeks after dermabrasion surgery.

Athletics

Strenuous athletic endeavors should be avoided for the first month. Exposure to *extremes* of heat, cold, or wind (as in snow skiing or other such outdoor sports) may damage the new skin and should be avoided for six months. The patient should remember to care for the new skin as carefully as that of a newborn.

It will gradually toughen and tolerate most of pre-dermabrasion activities.

POST-OPERATIVE VISITS

The patient will usually be seen by the physician the day following dermabrasion, and at several intervals for the next two weeks. The exact timing of these visits will vary from individual to individual, depending upon the healing process and the extent of the areas dermabraded. The patient should make every attempt to keep these appointments, since it is vitally important that the physician closely monitor the healing. If one lives in another city, the authors prefer a stay in town for several days after surgery. Depending upon the extent of the areas dermabraded, the authors may request that the patient stay at the hospital or clinic the night following surgery. Obviously, if small areas are dermabraded, one may be allowed to go directly home. Full-face dermabrasion patients may be asked to stay at the hospital or clinic for three to four days until it is certain the patient knows how to administer the post-operative instructions properly.

The patient should remember that swelling, crusting, and redness are expected with dermabrasion. One may be alarmed at the facial appearance for a week or so, patience is advised. Time and diligent skin care will help one to obtain the most favorable surgical result.

Close adherence to these instructions is vital to avoiding problems that might jeopardize the result.

The patient should notify the physician if he or she has any questions about the instructions or the healing process.

PART TWO

CHEMICAL PEEL

INTRODUCTION

Chemexfoliation (chemical peel) has been used to improve the texture of the skin since Sir Harold Gillies, an otolaryngologist, began using carbolic acid as an agent for eradication of increased elasticity of eyelid skin. Various agents have been used, including 20% resorcinol, salicylic acid, trichloroacetic acid (TCA), and B-naphthol. Ultraviolet light has also been used in an attempt to improve the texture of the skin; but as with the previously mentioned agents, it seems to affect only the superficial layers of the cutaneous structure. Phenol (carbolic acid), on the other hand, usually peels to a greater depth, and seems to produce more effective and consistent results than the other agents. In fact, this agent seems to be the most popular one used for chemical peel.

The senior author has used a modification of the technique described by Baker and Gordon for the past ten years. A similar chemical peel formula is used, but the McCollough technique eliminates taping, powdering, and crust formation. The results have been equally gratifying. Advantages of this technique include the omission of a second anesthetic for removal of the tape mask, reduced risk for post-operative scarring, and increased convenience and comfort for the patient.

CHEMISTRY OF THE PEEL SOLUTION

The peel formula is as follows:

1. Phenol 88%, U.S.P., 3 mL
2. Croton oil, 3 drops
3. Septisol Soap, 8 drops
4. Distilled water, 2 mL

In general, the depth of chemical peel is related to the strength and amount of the agent used. Paradoxically, more dilute solutions of phenol penetrate more deeply; therefore, it is wise not to alter the concentration of the formula.

Some clinicians believe that immediate occlusion with waterproof tape will increase the penetration of the peel solution. More than likely, the tape increases the degree of tissue maceration during the first two days, which alone produces additional tissue destruction (Fig. 44). It is the opinion of the authors that the application of a greater amount of the peel solution offsets any advantages of the tape mask used previously in this technique and others. In the authors' experience, the "maskless" method is effective and maintains a comfortable degree of safety.

The major active ingredient in the peel formula is phenol. Some believe that the concentrated form of phenol (greater than 80%) acts as a keratocoagulant by precipitating surface protein, and thus prevents penetration of the peel solution to the deeper layers of the skin. The concentration at which phenol transforms from a keratocoagulant to a keratolytic agent is not exactly known. It probably acts as a keratocoagulant in the formula, even though when mixed with the other components (e.g., croton oil, septisol, and water), its concentration is somewhat less than 80%. It has been noted that when the peel formula becomes diluted by tears, the initial insult appears deeper in the area of dilution, supporting the theory that the diluted form of phenol peels deeper.

The seed of Croton tiglium is composed of glycerides of several acids and a very toxic material: croton. Concentrated croton applied to the skin causes postular eruptions and skin destruction. Another component of the peel formula is a liquid soap, such as septisol, which is added to reduce surface tension and increase the penetration of phenol and croton oil more deeply into the keratin layers of the skin. Water is added to produce the "proper" chemical concentration of the emulsion.

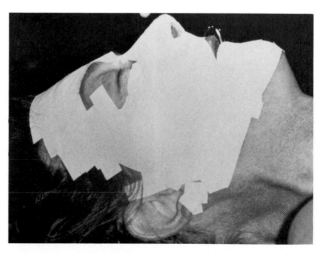

Figure 44. Tape mask used in "occlusive" technique. 53

As mentioned previously, precise mixture of the ingredients is important. A dependable and experienced assistant may prepare the solution. Some surgeons prefer to mix the ingredients themselves.

The preparation of the solution is begun with a small, clean, dry amber glass bottle, which should be labeled with the date and names or initials of the person(s) who actually prepared the formula. An additional safety factor is to have an assistant observing for confirmation of the accuracy of each step. A 3-mL syringe with an #18 gauge needle may be used to withdraw and accurately measure the phenol, which is then gently discharged into the amber glass bottle. If a smaller needle is used to extract the phenol, air may collect in the syringe under the negative pressure. A small glass dropper is then used to obtain and place the three drops of croton oil into the bottle. The same-sized dropper is used to obtain the eight drops of septisol soap. Finally, a 3- or 5-mL syringe is used to mix in the 2 mL of distilled water. The formula is capped and *safely* stored. The ingredients tend to settle out with standing. Vigorous mixing is required before use (Fig. 45).

The mixture of the ingredients of the peel formula is an emulsion. For this reason, it is wise to constantly agitate the contents in its container during the chemical peel procedure to ensure that proper concentration is maintained at the time of application. The solution is usually mixed fresh before each administration, but it can be stored in an amber glass bottled for short periods of time.

The peel formula is toxic in many ways. Phenol, in higher doses, can be hepatoxic, nephrotoxic, and cardiotoxic; therefore, the patient receiving this peel formula should be well hydrated before, during, and after its application.

When peeling more than one third of the face, the patient should have cardiac monitoring so that the

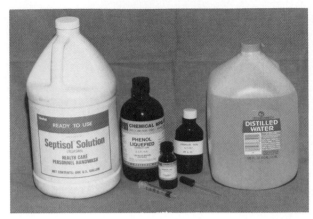

Figure 45. Septisol solution: Phenol 88%, U.S.P., croton oil, and distilled water. Exact portions are measured with a syringe and glass dropper. The mixture is placed in an amber glass bottle.

surgeon knows immediately if cardiac arrhythymas occur during the procedure.

If the peel solution is accidentally spilled onto an unintended area, one should quickly sponge the area covered by the excess amount of the peel solution to remove some of the solution before penetration. Glycerin may help prevent unwanted penetration in some cases.

If the peel solution is accidentally spilled into the eye, rapid irrigation with saline is recommended. This may seem contradictory, but it is a reasonable course of action. An ophthalmologic consultation is indicated should this unfortunate event occur.

Pooled tears in the medial and lateral canthal regions should be rapidly absorbed with cotton-tipped applicators. If tears come into contact with the peel solution, chemical diffusion and damage to the eye may follow. A trained assistant should be watching for tearing and mop them quickly.

8 Patient Selection

Table 3 lists the generally accepted indications for chemical peel.

Wrinkled, sun-damaged skin may respond well to a chemical face peel procedure. Not every patient with wrinkled facial skin, however, is a candidate for chemical peel. In general, the thin-skinned female with a fair complexion and fine rhytids is a good candidate. A fair complexion may help camouflage any color contrast at the margins of the treated areas (Fig. 46).

Dark-skinned individuals, on the other hand, are more likely to demonstrate pigmentary changes, since the peel solution produces some degree of hypopigmentation in almost all cases.

Superficial pigmentated lesions, such as lentigo, may be improved at least for awhile; but in many cases, they do not always respond to the chemical face peel procedure. Freckles may disappear for a few months only to reappear later. This is not to say that chemical peel is contraindicated in treating freckles. In fact, the authors have had good results in treating this condition (Fig. 47).

Isolated seborrheic keratoses may also be eradicated, or at least improved, by chemical peel but are probably better treated by simple curratage. If the entire face is affected by these and other undesirable signs of aging and sun damage, a full face peel combined with superficial curratage is helpful (see Fig. 24).

Superficial acne scars may be improved following chemical peel. Deep acne scarring, on the other hand, is minimally improved, if at all, by this procedure. We feel that deep scars are much better treated by a combination of dermabrasion and/or punch grafting.

As with dermabrasion, before surgery, patients should understand that the color of the skin in the treated areas will be altered by chemical peel. Most females have no problem coping with the altered skin tones because these areas may be covered with makeup. Males, on the other hand, may have more difficulty camouflaging color differentials because most do not wear makeup. Nevertheless, the authors have had excellent results peeling many male patients.

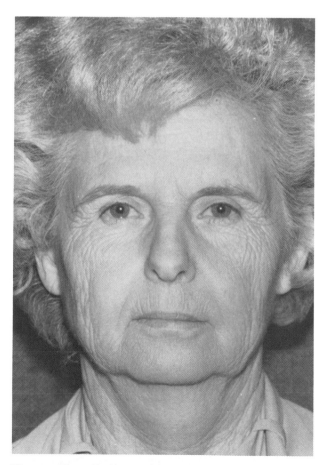

Figure 46a. Patient with wrinkled, sun-damaged skin. Thin skin and fair complexion help make this patient a good candidate for chemical peel.

Table 3. Indications for Chemical Peel

Wrinkled, sun-damaged skin (rhytids)
Lentigo
Keratosis (seborrheic or actinic)
Superficial acne
In combination with facial rejuvenation procedures

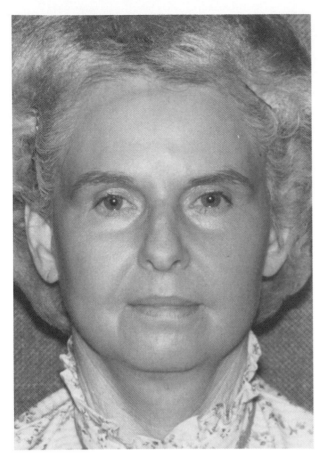

Figure 46b.   Post-chemical peel.

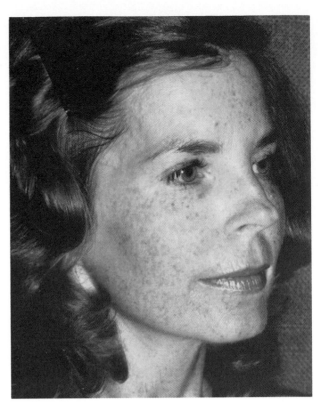

Figure 47b.   Right oblique view.

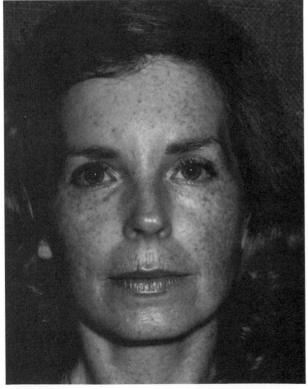

Figure 47a.   Patient with freckling (antero-posterior view).

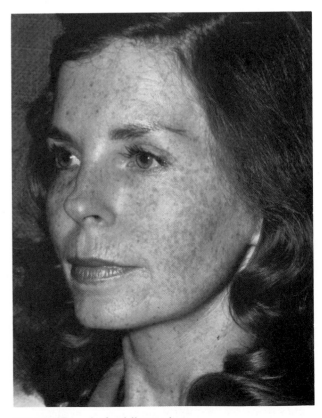

Figure 47c.   Left oblique view.

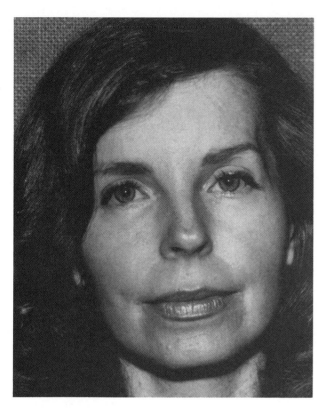

Figure 47d. Post-chemical peel (antero-posterior view).

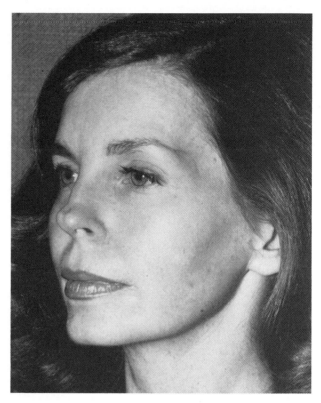

Figure 47f. Left oblique view.

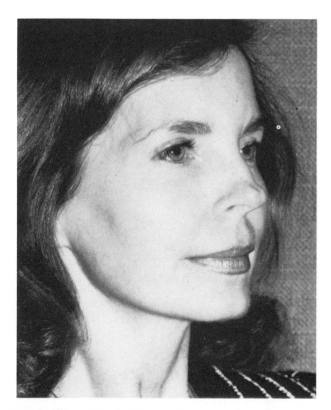

Figure 47e. Right oblique view.

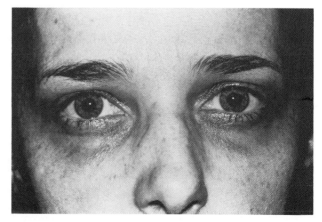

Figure 47g. Patient with periorbital hyperpigmentation.

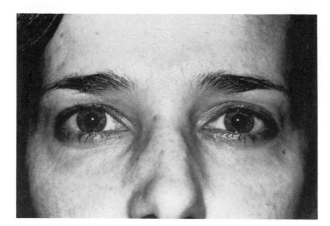

Figure 47h.   Post-chemical peel.

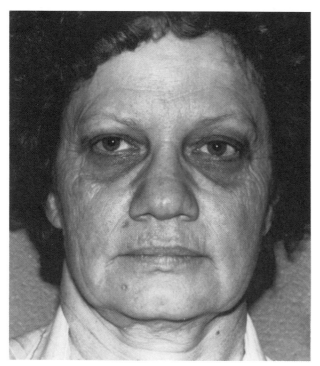

Figure 47i.   Patient with periorbital hyperpigmentation (antero-posterior view).

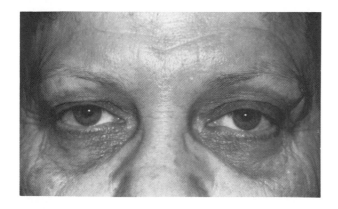

Figure 47j.   Periorbital close-up view.

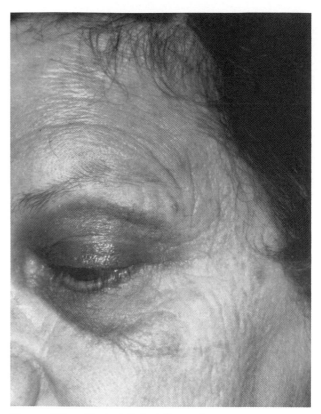

Figure 47k.   Periorbital oblique view.

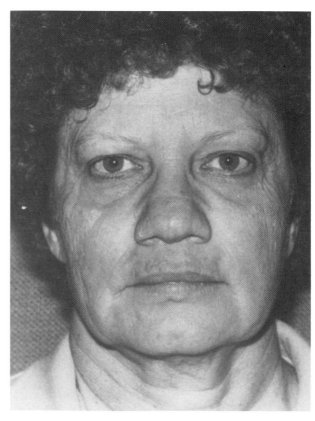

Figure 47l.   Six weeks post-peel (antero-posterior view).

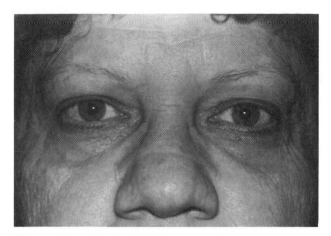

Figure 47m. Periorbital close-up view.

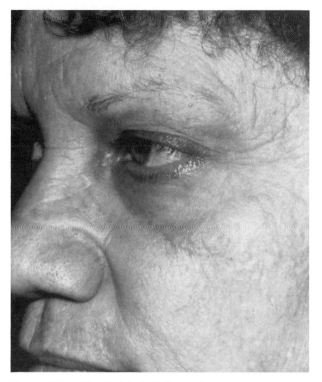

Figure 47n. Periorbital oblique view.

9　Pre-Operative Considerations

Pre-operative photographs are recommended. The following views are taken: full face, lateral, and oblique. In special areas of consideration, such as the periorbital or perioral regions, close-up photographs may be taken.

Printed materials informing the patient about the procedure and pre- and post-operative periods are usually provided for the patient before the initial consultation. The patient is asked to study this material and write down any questions. During the consultation interview, the factors pertaining to the patients problem, the procedure, and the healing period are reviewed. In addition, the patient is offered an opportunity to inquire about the alternative methods of treatment and the potential risks, limitations, complications, and possibility of any additional surgical procedures that might be required. On the day of the procedure, the above factors are reviewed once again.

In the pre-operative period, it is especially important that the patient understand how terrible he or she will look within the first few days following the procedure. Even after the surgeon's best attempt to explain the expected immediate post-operative appearance, many patients and/or family members are unpleasantly surprised (Fig. 48).

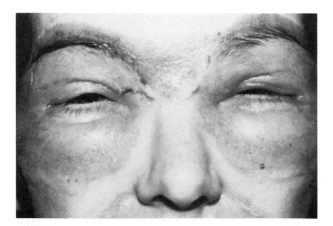

Figure 48. Patients may experience significant post-operative swelling. This patient is 19 hours post-periorbital peel.

In the authors' practice, chemical peel is usually performed in an outpatient setting. On the morning of surgery, the patient's face is washed three times with septisol soap. (pHisoderm® may leave a film that could interfere with the penetration of the peel components.) The patient should thoroughly rinse away the soap before the procedure. Pre-operatively, the patient is usually given oral doses of 250 mg tetracycline, 20 mg Valium®, 200 mg Dramamine®, and 40 mg prednisone.

Before initiation of "twilight" sleep, the patient is taken to the operating suite, where an intravenous line is inserted. Most patients are given 0.10 mg (0.25 cc) scopolamine intravenously. If less than one third of the patient's face is to be peeled, the only medications given may be two buffered aspirin and two acetaminophen-hydrocodone tablets.

Patients undergoing full-face peels are connected to a cardiac monitor. It is advisable to have resuscitative equipment and medications available in case dangerous cardiac arrhythmias occur. Although the authors have observed cardiac arrhythymias in some patients, cardiovascular decompensation requiring the use of resuscitative or supportive measures has never been encountered. After the pre-operative medications have taken effect and the cardiac monitor and intravenous line have been connected to the patient, local anesthetic field blocks and infiltration are performed. If the peel procedure is restricted to a single aesthetic unit, an anesthetic mixture including equal parts of Marcaine® (bupivacaine Hcl) (0.25%) and lidocaine (1%) without epinephrine is used. If, on the other hand, a full-face peel is to be performed, the same combination to anesthetize the forehead is used; plain Marcaine® (0.25%) can be used to anesthetize the remainder of the face. In the authors' experience, this routine significantly reduces pain during the procedure and the post-operative period.

The patient may feel *some* burning when the peel is applied, even though local anesthetics have been used. Intravenous Valium®, in 2.5-mg increments, is given every five to ten minutes, as needed, during application of the local anesthesia to keep the patient comfortable. The total intravenous Valium® dose is generally restricted to 20 mg. Some patients have a high tolerance to sedatives, tranquilizers, and hypnotics. If additional relaxation is required, 0.5 mg hydromorphone may be used.

The areas to be peeled are thoroughly cleansed with an acetone-dampened 2 X 2 inch sponge, folded and grasped with a hemostat (Fig. 49). The acetone is applied repeatedly until a sandpaper-like sound is heard as the sponge is rubbed across the skin. At this point, most of the oily substances will have been removed, and the face is ready for the application of the peel solution. Without the removal of the natural surface oils, the peel may not penetrate to the proper depth, and the patient could be left with "skip areas" and a less than satisfactory result. This step in the procedure is as important as any that may follow. Ether has been used by some surgeons to clean the oily substances from the skin's surface, but the authors prefer the use of the less flammable acetone.

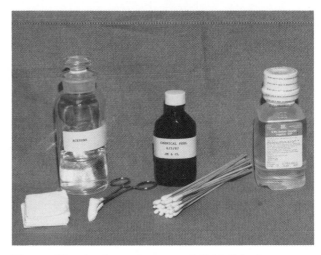

Figure 49. Acetone-dampened 2 X 2 inch sponge folded over a hemostat is used to remove facial oils from the region(s) to be peeled. Cotton-tipped applicators are used to apply the mixture, which is kept in an amber glass bottle. Sterile saline should be available (via a large syringe or irrigation bottle) in case of accidental occular exposure. Dry cotton-tipped applicators are also used to mop periorbital tearing.

10   Procedure

When performing a full-face peel, the solution should be applied carefully and precisely to the six aesthetic facial units (see drawing). If a full-face peel is to be performed, the procedure is begun first on the forehead unit. A wooden-handled, cotton-tipped applicator is dipped into the amber glass bottle containing the peel solution, as the surgical assistant constantly moves the glass bottle to keep the emulsion mixed. Before the applicator is removed from the bottle, the cotton head is gently rolled against the inside of the glass bottle to squeeze any excess peel solution from the cotton. Neither the bottle nor the applicator stick should ever be passed over the patient's eyes. When the forehead is peeled, the surgeon and the assistant holding the amber bottle stand at the head of the patient, cephalic to the eyes. Likewise, when the lower face or lower eyelids are peeled, the surgeon as well as the assistant with the amber bottle stand caudal to an imaginary horizontal plane passing through the eyes (Fig. 50).

The procedure begins by rolling the moistened, cotton-tipped applicator across the skin of patient's forehead. The solution is feathered into the hair-

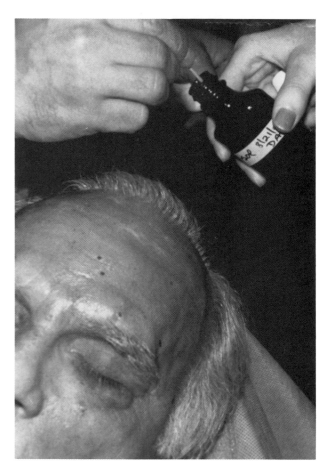

Figure 50. When peeling the forehead, the surgeon and the assistant stand cephalic to the patient's eyes to ensure no liquid passes across the eyes. (Photo courtesy of Dr. Daniel Russo.)

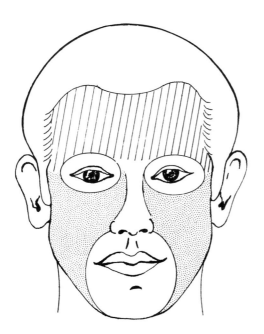

bearing areas of the forehead hair, sideburns, and eyebrows. This tends to prevent a sharp demarcation at the edge of the treated regions. Intravenous fluids (usually D5W) are allowed to flow at approximately 500 cc/h during the peel procedure. The authors generally wait about 10 to 15 minutes, while observing the cardiac monitor, between peeling aesthetic units (Fig. 51).

Next, the right cheek is peeled. After a 10 to 15 minute observation period, the left cheek is peeled. Care should be taken to feather the solution into the

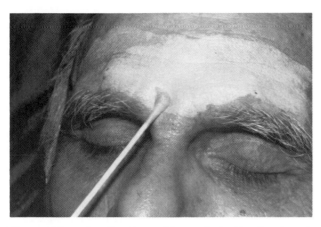

Figure 51a. Application of formula to the forehead. The moistened applicator is rolled over the region being treated. (Photo courtesy of Dr. Daniel Russo.)

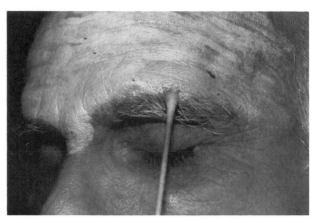

Figure 51d. Feathering onto the superior portion of the brow. (Photo courtesy of Dr. Daniel Russo.)

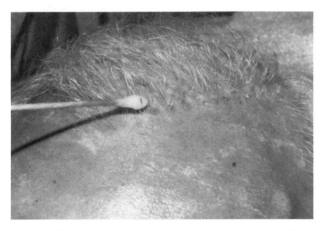

Figure 51b. Feathering onto the frontal hairline. This patient is also undergoing hair replacement. (Photo courtesy of Dr. Daniel Russo.)

sideburns, as well as over the angle of the mandible. One should be careful not to peel too far onto the neck (Fig. 52).

After both cheeks have been peeled, the next aesthetic unit treated is the perioral area. When peeling around the mouth, one must be careful to feather the peel over onto the pink vermillion of the lips. If this is not done, a demarcation line may be left around the perioral edge at the vermillion border. If the lips contain deep rhytids, the frayed, broken wooden edge of a dry, unused applicator stick may be used to apply small portions of the peel into the deep grooves (Fig. 53).

The next aesthetic unit treated is the periorbital area. First, we will discuss the lower eyelids. When peeling this area, the surgeon and the assistant stand below the patient's eyes so that no peel solution could be dropped into the eyes.

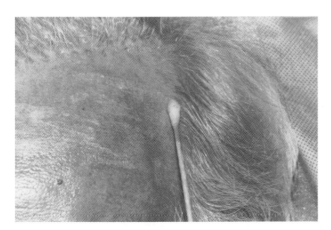

Figure 51c. Feathering the lateral hairline. (Photo courtesy of Dr. Daniel Russo.)

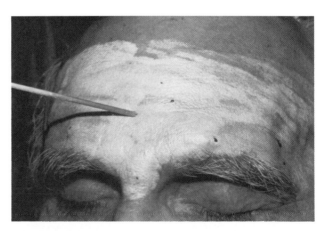

Figure 51e. The frayed wooden end of an applicator may be used to apply extra peel solution to deeper creases. (Photo courtesy of Dr. Daniel Russo.)

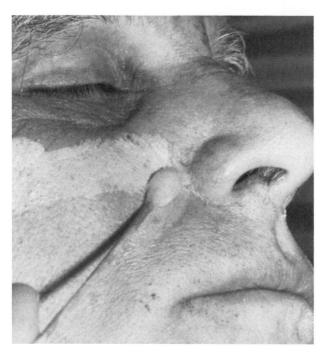

Figure 52a. Application of formula to the cheeks. (Photo courtesy of Dr. Daniel Russo.)

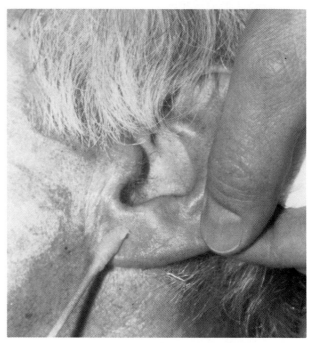

Figure 52c. Peeling may be carried just onto the lobule of the ear to help blend the treated and untreated areas. (Photo courtesy of Dr. Daniel Russo.)

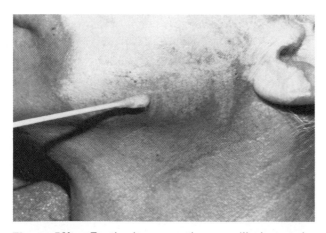

Figure 52b. Feathering over the mandibular angle. One should be cautious not to peel down onto the neck. (Photo courtesy of Dr. Daniel Russo.)

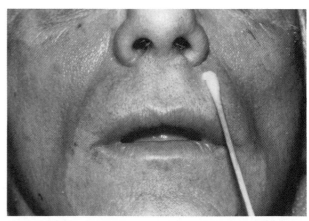

Figure 53a. Application of the peel solution to the perioral region. Again, the moistened applicator is rolled over the skin surface. (Photo courtesy of Dr. Daniel Russo.)

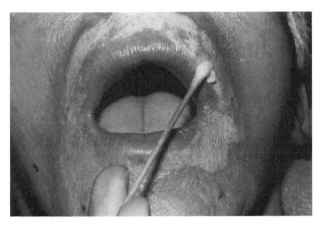

Figure 53b. The peel is carried 2 to 3 mm onto the vermillion of the lips. (Photo courtesy of Dr. Daniel Russo.)

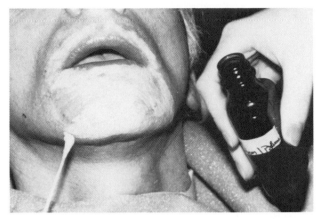

Figure 53d. The entire perioral region and chin is treated. Feathering is gently carried over the mandibular margin. (Photo courtesy of Dr. Daniel Russo.)

The cotton-tipped applicator is dipped and partially dried against the inside edge of the bottle. It is wise to have the applicator a little dryer when peeling the periorbital region. The patient is asked to look superiorly to help tighten the lower lid skin. The peel solution is applied to the lower eyelid to within 2 to 3 mm of the lid margin. An assistant should be standing by with a bottle of sterile saline to immediately irrigate the eye if any peel solution comes into contact with the eye. In addition, the assistants should be ready with *dry,* cotton-tipped applicators to mop any tearing that may occur. Tearing may allow some of the chemicals to diffuse in a retrograde manner into the eye. If tearing is allowed to flow onto the peeled area, the solution may become diluted, enhancing the keratolytic effect and penetrating too deeply.

When peeling the upper eyelids, the patient is asked to close the eyes. The surgeon and assistant stand cephalic to the eyes. The upper eyelid is likewise peeled to within 2 to 3 mm of the lid margin. Again,

careful attention must be maintained to mop any tearing that occurs at the medial and lateral canthal regions. If there is redundancy of the upper lid skin, the brow should be lifted to tighten the skin during the application of the peel, so that it is applied evenly to all of the upper lid skin (Fig. 54). Generally, any nasal peeling (Fig. 55) is done last.

While applying the peel solution, one will note the immediate development of a white frost—providing, of course, the treated areas have been adequately cleaned and the surface oils properly removed with acetone. Upon application of the peel solution, the patient will experience an immediate stinging or burning sensation, which disappears within seconds.

One should extend the peel solution into the hair-bearing areas of the brows and scalp. The authors have not observed any hair loss from this procedure. Failure to feather the peel into the hair may leave an obvious line of demarcation.

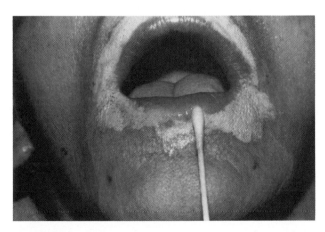

Figure 53c. The peel is carried 2 to 3 mm onto the vermillion of the lips. (Photo courtesy of Dr. Daniel Russo.)

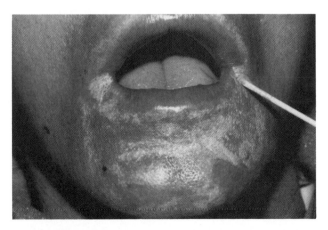

Figure 53e. Small amounts of extra peel solution may be applied to the deep rhytids. (Photo courtesy of Dr. Daniel Russo.)

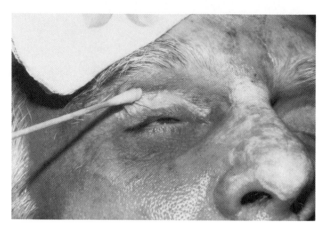

Figure 54a. The eyes are closed and the brow lifted to tighten any redundant skin when peeling the upper eyelid. (Photo courtesy of Dr. Daniel Russo.)

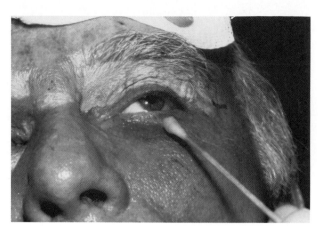

Figure 54c. When peeling the lower eyelid, the patient looks superiorly to help tighten the eyelid skin. The peel is carried to within 2 to 3 mm of the eyelid margin. (Photo courtesy of Dr. Daniel Russo.)

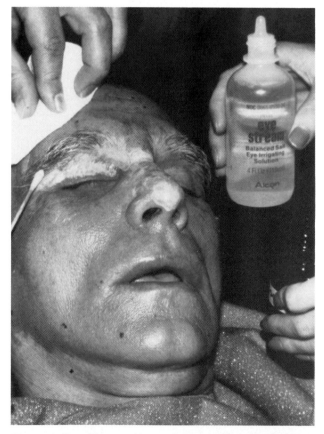

Figure 54b. The peel is carried to within 2 to 3 mm of the eyelid margin. Feathering is also carried up onto the lower portion of the eyebrow. Saline irrigation is ready in case of an accidental spill. Clean-dry cotton-tipped applicators are used to dry any tearing. (Photo courtesy of Dr. Daniel Russo.)

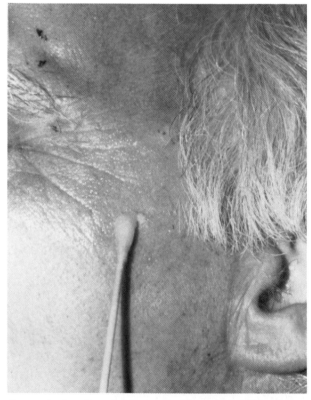

Figure 54d. The lateral periorbital area is treated to improve the "crow's feet." (Photo courtesy of Dr. Daniel Russo.)

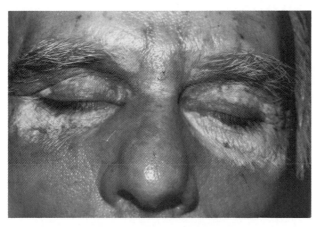

Figure 54e. After treatment of the entire periorbital region, blending has been accomplished to all peripheral areas (brow, lateral periorbital, etc.) The lid margins are untreated. (Photo courtesy of Dr. Daniel Russo.)

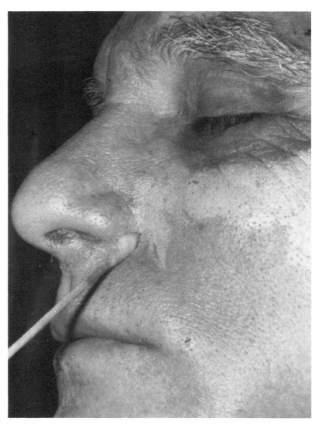

Figure 55b. Feathering is performed as necessary, and the alar facial groove is treated. (Photo courtesy of Dr. Daniel Russo.)

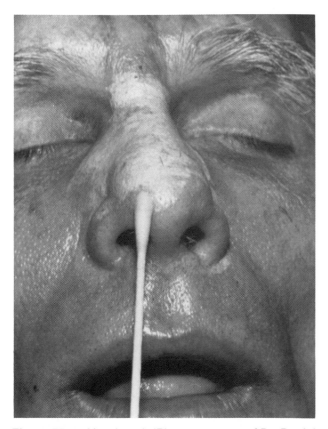

Figure 55a. Nasal peel. (Photo courtesy of Dr. Daniel Russo.)

11   Post-Operative Considerations

The usual post-operative medications include 250 mg tetracycline q.i.d., multivitamins q.d., 5 mg Valium® h.s. as needed, and acetaminophen-oxycodone or (hydrocodone) every four hours as needed for pain. Aspirin is an excellent analgesic for the type of discomfort associated with chemical peel.

After completion of the procedure, the intravenous line is maintained and D5W is administered for approximately two hours at a rate of 500 cc/h. After this period, the cardiac monitor may be removed and intravenous fluids are continued at 100 cc/h for an additional two hours.

About 20 minutes after the peel application and the disappearance of the initial stinging, the pain should return. Many patients have described this as a burning-type pain. After shorter-acting local anesthetics wear off, this pain may become fairly significant. Acetaminophen-hydrocodone and/or aspirin is usually sufficient to make the patient reasonably comfortable. During the first six to seven hours post-operatively, the patient may require stronger analgesics. Occasionally, several acetaminophen-hydrocodone tablets along with aspirin may be required. Analgesics are titrated for patient comfort. After about eight hours, the pain generally disappears and does not recur.

The morning after the procedure, many patients claim they experience none of the painful, burning pain they had during the first hours after surgery. They may, however, have some discomfort of a lesser degree. This may be associated with edema and the desquamation process of the superficial layers of the skin.

During the first post-operative day, the skin will become very edematous and gray in color. The first signs of desquamation are apparent at this time. The most significant observation to the patient who has had a periorbital peel is that the eyes may sometimes be swollen shut. After a perioral peel, some patients experience a fairly significant protrusion of the lips. Other areas are simply edematous and discolored (Fig. 56). Although the patient has been informed pre-operatively of what to expect, he or she will need to be reassured upon seeing the swelling and discoloration on the first post-operative day. The condi-

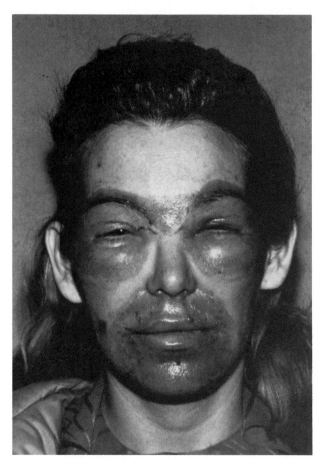

Figure 56a. Significant periorbital and perioral swelling 19 hours post-operatively.

tion may actually worsen by the second post-operative day; but after the third and fourth day, the swelling begins to subside, and the desquamating skin begins to slough. The immediate post-operative appearance and the residual effects of the operative medications may cause the patient to be depressed. Patience and encouragement are helpful if this should occur (Fig. 57).

All of the desquamated skin and crusting is usually shed by seven to ten days, and the skin appears very erythematous by this time.

On the day after surgery, the patient is instructed to begin showering six times daily, after which he or

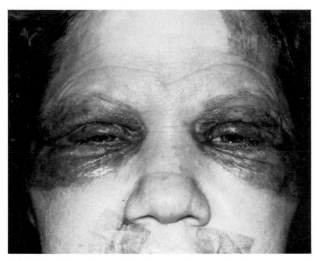

Figure 56b. Periorbital swelling 22 hours post-operatively.

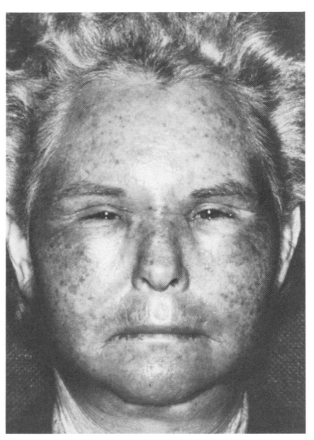

Figure 57a. Swelling one day post-operatively (see Fig. 46a).

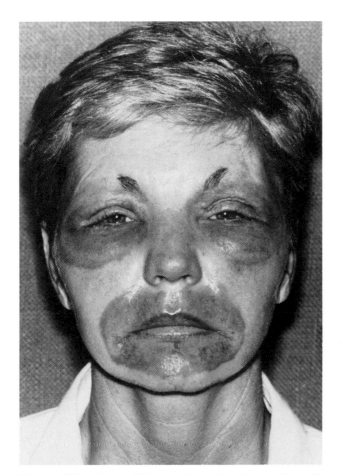

Figure 56c. Periorbital and perioral swelling 21 hours post-operatively.

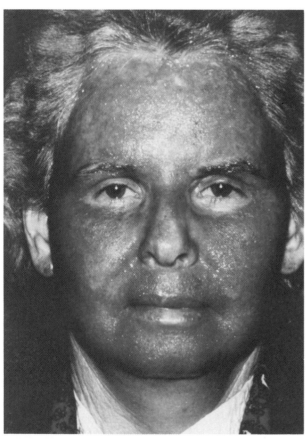

Figure 57b.   Appearance five days post-operatively.

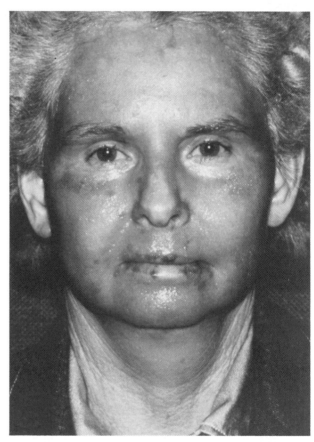

Figure 57c.   Appearance nine days post-operatively. Also note the development of herpetic erruptions.

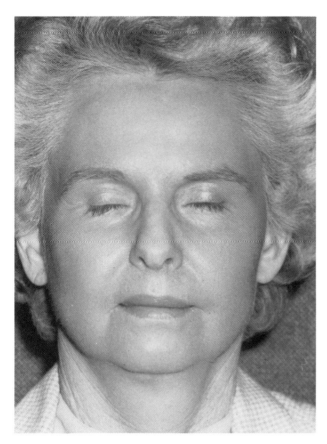

Figure 57d. Appearance 17 days post-operatively.

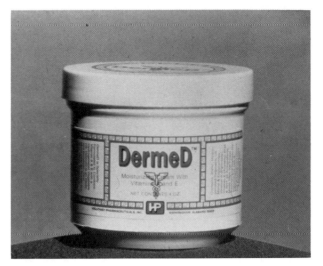

Figure 58. Dermed® cream.

she is to cover the peeled areas with a thick layer of a vegetable oil-based cream (Dermed® or Crisco® solid shortening) (Fig. 58). After the initial desquamation is completed (10 to 14 days), the patient can often begin to wear a water-based makeup, if they desire. Patients, however, are asked to wait until they have been examined in the clinic before applying makeup.

The new healing skin is very delicate, especially in the initial stage. The patient is instructed not to pick any desquamating skin from the cheeks. Any crusting is removed by repeated tepid water washings and the application of creams that soften and lubricate the skin. They allow the crust to be shed naturally. If the desquamating skin is plucked away, it is possible to convert a second-degree defect into a third-degree defect, which could result in scarring.

As with dermabrasion, the intense pink color that is apparent after the initial healing stage gradually fades over the next 8 to 12 weeks. The patient should be instructed to avoid direct sunlight for at least six months post-operatively to avoid damaging the sensitive new skin. Exposure to sunlight during this critical period may result in hyperpigmentation. The patient is also instructed to use at least sun protection factor #15 sunscreens when exposed to any sun. This is not to imply that patients may expose their skin to sunlight if they wear the sunscreen. It is used as an *added* protection. Direct sunlight should be avoided during this initial healing period.

For several weeks after surgery, the patient may need to use moisturizing creams at night to keep the new skin from drying. Most patients can return to work at the end of the second post-operative week as long as they are not involved in outdoor activities that would subject them to sunlight, heat, cold, or wind.

12   Contraindications

CONTRAINDICATIONS TO CHEMICAL PEEL

Table 4 lists the contraindications to chemical peel. The dark-skinned patient is generally not an ideal candidate for a deep chemical face peel procedure. Post-operative pigmentary abnormalities may be more likely to occur. Since the skin is usually expected to be somewhat lighter after this procedure, there would be greater discrepancies in skin color between the peeled and nonpeeled areas. It is also possible that various shades of spotty, pigmentary aberrations may be more apparent on the dark-skinned patient.

Skin of the Neck

One may run the risk of hypertrophic scar formation if the neck skin is peeled (see the section on "Complications"). Although the authors feather over the angle of the mandible when performing a full face peel, one should be careful not to peel too far down onto the neck skin.

Renal, Hepatic, Cardiac Disease

One should exercise caution when peeling patients with renal, hepatic, or cardiac disease due to the phenol component of the peel formula. If a patient has significant problems with any of these organ systems, one should consider obtaining a medical consultation. The authors' pre-operative workup includes studies that may uncover an abnormality in the liver or kidney of the patient who has a negative history. Since epinephrine can exacerbate cardiac arrhythmias, it is probably wise not to use an epinephrine-containing local anesthetic.

Active Herpetic Lesions

If the patient has a history of Herpes labialis (fever blisters), there is a high likelihood that a chemical peel procedure will cause an exacerbation of these lesions post-operatively. One may proceed with a chemical peel procedure after explaining this possibility to the patient, and having provided a prescription for Zovirax® (acyclovir). The patient who contracts herpetic lesions (fever blisters) during the healing process could experience a spread of these lesions over the entire area that has been peeled. For this reason, patients treat the entire area with oral and topical Zovirax® until healing is complete.

Use of Hormonal Medications

Some surgeons believe that estrogen and progesterone may contribute to post-operative pigmentary changes. It may be important for patients to abstain from any hormonal replacement therapy or birth control pills for at least six months post-operatively.

The Unrealistic or Unreliable Patient

Contraindications also include the unrealistic or unreliable patient. The patient should have a clear understanding of the procedure, post-operative care, and

---

Table 4.   Relative Contraindications for Chemical Peel

Active herpetic lesions (fever blisters)
Use of hormonal medications (e.g., estrogen, progesterone)
Unrealistic patient expectations
Unreliable patient
Skin of the neck
Renal disease*
Hepatic disease*
Cardiac disease*
Epinephrine-containing local anesthetic—exercise caution when performed in conjunction with associated surgery (e.g., regional perioral peel with face lift)

*A medical consultation should be obtained.

post-operative appearance. The patient must be mature enough to accept the immediate post-operative swelling and change in appearance, which are part of the process one must go through to achieve the desired result. The patient should also understand that some degree of pigmentary change is expected in exchange for a smoother, younger-looking skin. The patient must be realistic about what can be achieved. In addition, the patient must be willing to follow the post-operative instructions very closely, and understand one must avoid the sun for at least six months post-operatively.

Post-operative instructions for patients who have had a chemical peel are discussed in Chapter 14.

13   Complications

Cardiac arrhythmias have been known to occur during the cutaneous application of phenol. Phenol is slowly excreted from the kidneys. The chemical peel procedure, therefore, requires cardiac monitoring, as well as adequate hydration with intravenous fluids. Premature atrial contractions, premature ventricular contractions, bigeminy, and trigeminy may occur within minutes after the use of phenol if the patient is overly sensitive, or if more than one-third of the face is peeled within a 10- to 15-minute period. If arrhythmias occur, application of the peel should be stopped until normal sinus rhythm has returned for a full 15 minutes. Then the procedure may be resumed; but one may be well advised to extend the intervals between peeling the aesthetic units for an additional 15 minutes.

If no arrhythmias occur, this procedure may take about 90 minutes to peel an entire face, allowing 15 minutes between each of the aesthetic regions peeled (forehead, right cheek, left cheek, perioral, periorbital, and nasal regions).

Exacerbation of lesions sometimes occurs in the perioral regions in patients who carry the Herpes simplex virus. For patients with a history of fever blisters (see section on "Active Herpetic Lesions"), the authors often recommend 200 mg Zovirax® orally every four hours before the procedure; this should be continued for six to seven days into the post-operative period. It is advisable not to perform a peel procedure on a patient who has an *active* fever blister. A high percentage of patients with a history of facial Herpes eruptions will exhibit an exacerbation, especially around the mouth. If this should occur in the post-operative period, Zovirax® treatment is begun as described; in addition, topical Zovirax® ointment may be used. The authors have not observed any permanent skin defects in the areas of the Herpes lesions (Fig. 59).

Prophylactic antiviral ointments may be applied into the eyes of patients who carry the Herpes virus and who are undergoing a chemical peel procedure. In the authors' experience, this has not been necessary; no ocular complications have been observed.

If pigmentary aberrations are going to occur, they usually become evident within three to six months post-operatively. In fair-skinned individuals, demar-

cation lines between the peeled and nonpeeled areas are less of a problem. The feathering technique is used at the borders of treated and nontreated areas, such as the angle of the jaw, hair-bearing areas, and the vermillion border of the lips. When regional peels are performed, it is especially important to feather into the surrounding areas.

In some cases, hyperpigmentation may occur or reappear in previously pigmented regions. A cream composed of 15 g Eldoquin Forte® (hydroquinone 4%) and 15 g (0.1%) Retin A (retinoic acid) may help. One could start with once daily applications and increase or decrease as tolerated.

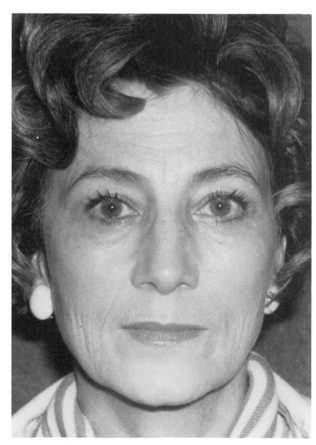

Figure 59a.   Pre-operative patient with a history of fever blisters (antero-posterior view).

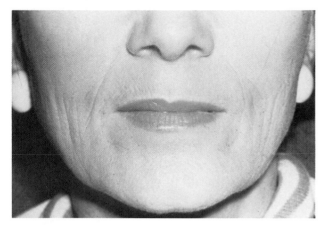

Figure 59b. Close-up view.

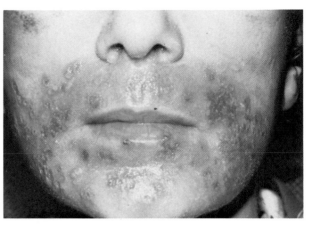

Figure 59d. Perioral close-up view.

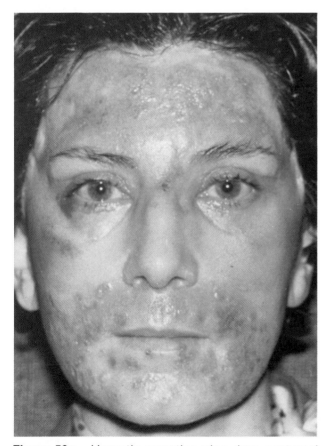

Figure 59c. Herpetic erruption nine days post-peel (antero-posterior view).

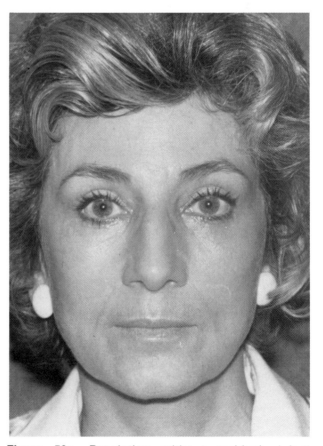

Figure 59e. Resolution without residual defect (antero-posterior view).

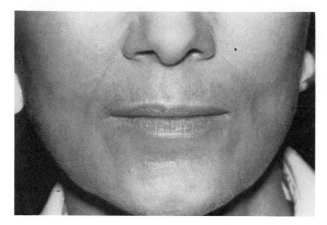

Figure 59f.   Perioral close-up view.

The tendency to develop hyperpigmentation may be exacerbated if the patient is exposed to sunlight or is taking estrogen- or progesterone-containing medications; or if the patient becomes pregnant within the first six months post-procedure.

Occasionally, an uneven application of the peel or peeling over areas that have not been adequately cleaned with acetone may cause spotty hyperpigmentation. If this occurs, hyperpigmented areas can be touched up or repeeled in about three months. On the other hand, hypopigmentation is more commonly seen, and is expected after a peel procedure. It is not considered a complication, but an expected side effect after a successful peel (Fig. 60).

Lentigenes can occasionally be removed with the chemical peel procedure. In many cases, the hyperpigmented areas will return. The response of these lentigenes to chemical peel is directly related to the depth of the melanocytes. It makes sense that if the melanin deposits are very deep, then the freckles will return. It is for this reason the authors try to inform patients that the removal of freckles is somewhat unpredictable. The authors will attempt the procedure if the patient accepts these uncertainties.

In hypersensitive patients, erythema may persist beyond the three-month period. If this occurs, the patient should be reassured that time will most likely correct this problem (2.5% hydrocortisone cream may help). The patient should be informed, however, that the peeled skin will be different in color and texture from the nonpeeled areas, and that this could be a permanent change. The patient should be prepared to accept pigmentary irregularities in exchange for the smoother and more youthful-looking skin. Women can camouflage these areas with makeup if necessary.

Hypertrophic scarring very rarely occurs. It is most likely to occur along the mandible margins or in the perioral region. The authors treated one patient who

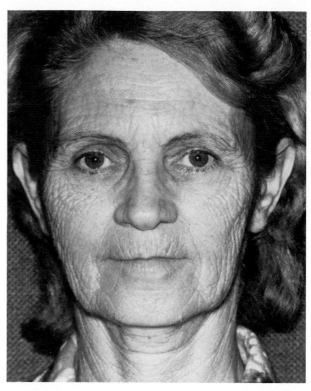

Figure 60a.   Patient before a face lift, eyelid surgery, and chemical peel procedures (antero-posterior view).

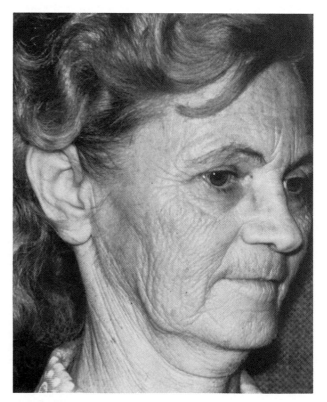

Figure 60b.   Oblique view.

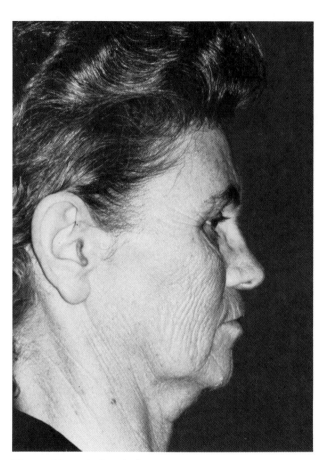

Figure 60c.   Lateral view.

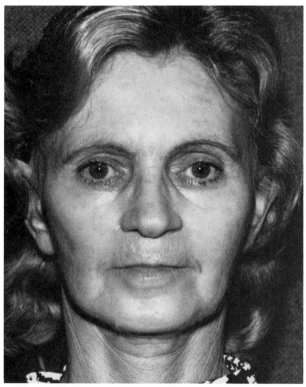

Figure 60d. After face lift, eyelid, and chemical peel procedures. There is some degree of post-peel hypopigmentation in this fair-skinned patient. This may be a side effect exchanged for smoother skin (antero-posterior view).

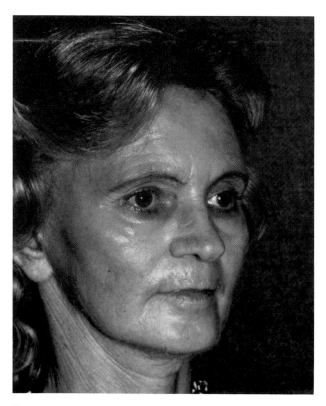

Figure 60e. Oblique view.

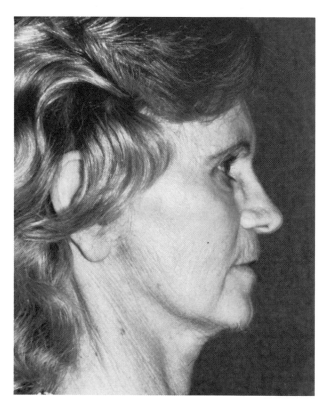

Figure 60f. Lateral view.

experienced some scarring on the forehead along the hairline, where she wore a shower cap with a tight headband in the immediate post-operative period. The pressure in this area converted a second-degree defect to a third-degree wound. Fortunately, adequate local treatment made any residual defect nearly imperceptible. If hypertrophic scarring occurs, these areas can be treated with Kenalog® (triamcinolone) (10 or 20 mg/cc) injections until resolved. If a scar does not completely heal within six months, one may consider excision. Fortunately, the authors have not had to deal with this situation. If hypertrophic scarring does occur, the use of intralesional steroids, patient support, and time should solve the problem.

The senior author has been consulted on cases of severe hypertrophic scarring resulting from a procedure known as exodermatology, performed elsewhere in which formulas other than those commonly recommended and a tape mask were used (Figs. 61, 62).

Wound infections are extremely rare after a chemical peel procedure as long as the patient faithfully follows the post-operative cleaning instructions. The senior author treated one elderly patient who developed a full-face *Pseudomonas* infection as a result of not showering or cleansing the face for several days. After the situation was discovered, the patient was vigorously cleaned, and the infection resolved. She obtained an excellent result (Fig. 63).

Milia may occur within the first four to six weeks post-operatively. These lesions usually subside with a normal cleansing regimen. If this fails, however, a #18 gauge needle can be used to uncap the epidermal inclusion cyst; healing will soon follow.

Subtotal removal of facial rhytids should not be considered a complication. Some rhytids cannot be removed. Subtotal removal may be the result of insufficient application of the chemical peel formula, inadequate removal of facial oils, or simply deep rhytids

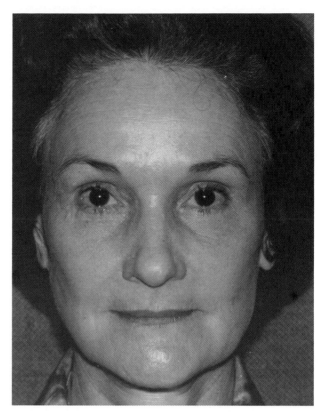

Figure 61b. This patient was consulted and photographed before going to another center for peeling (antero-posterior view).

that require additional peeling. Perfection rarely follows any plastic surgical procedure. Repeeling may be necessary. Additional improvement may be obtained in many cases. The deep forehead lines and nasolabial folds cannot be removed by chemical peel. The patient should be informed of this fact before the chemical peel procedure.

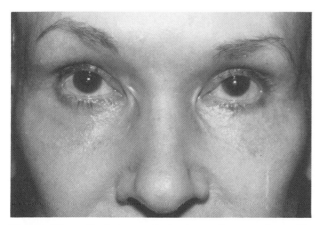

Figure 61a. Patient peeled at another center with exodermatology and taping. Medial canthal scarring is shown.

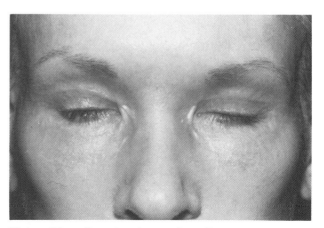

Figure 61c. Scarring (eyes closed).

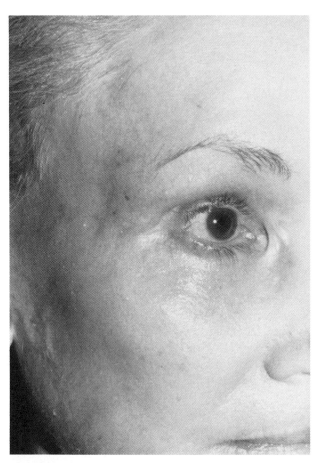

Figure 61d. Scarring (periorbital oblique view).

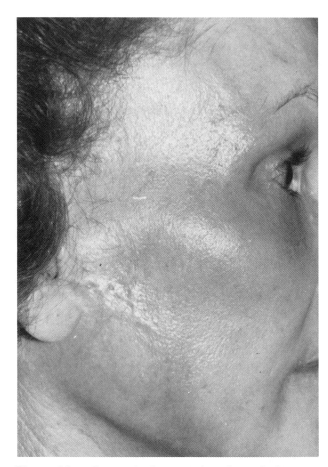

Figure 61e. Pre-auricular scarring (lateral close-up view).

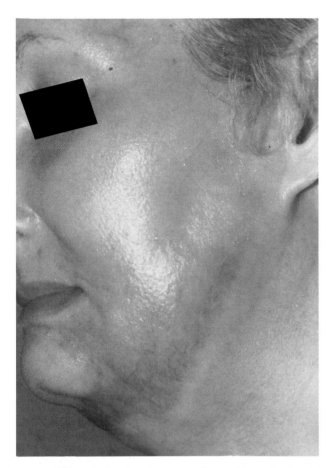

Figure 62a. Patient referred to the authors for treatment of neck scarring after exodermatology.

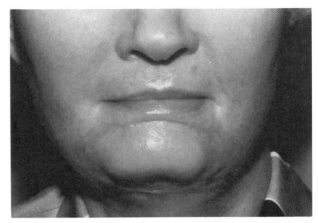

Figure 62c. Chin and submental scarring.

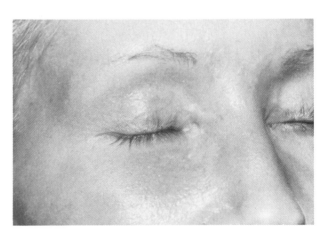

Figure 62d. Medial canthal scarring.

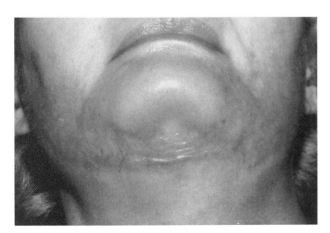

Figure 62b. Submental scarring.

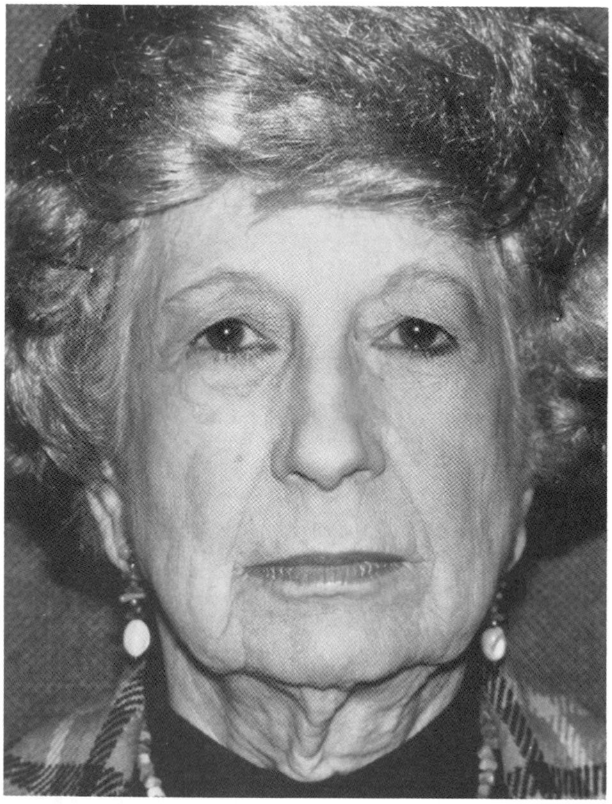

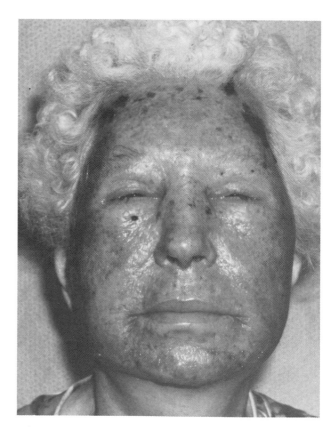

Figure 63a. Patient who failed to follow post-operative cleaning instructions; pre-operative face lift, blepharoplasty, and chemical peel.

Figure 63b. One day post-peel; significant swelling.

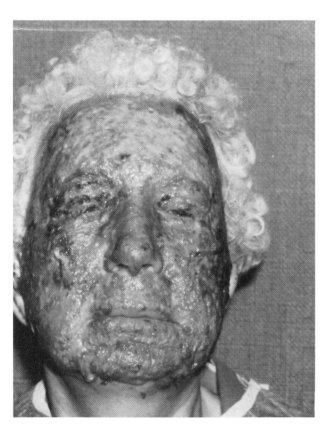

Figure 63c. Fourth day post-peel; patient has not followed cleaning instructions and has a full-face infection.

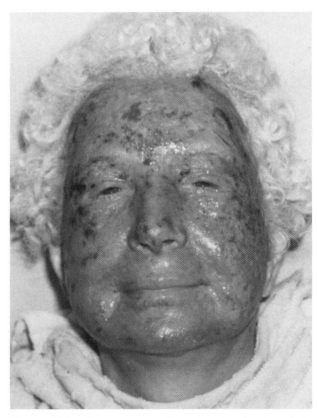

Figure 63d. Appearance after cleaning in the clinic on the fourth day post-operatively.

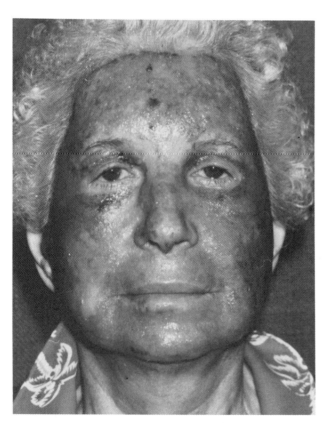

Figure 63e.   One week post-operatively.

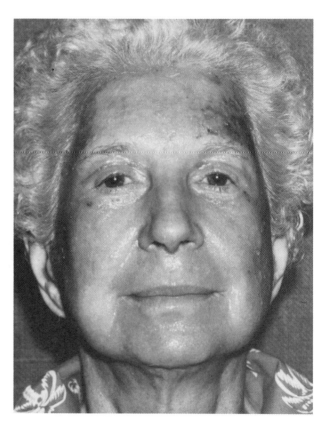

Figure 63f. Two weeks and two days post-operatively.

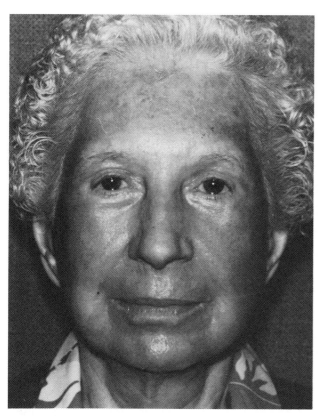

Figure 63g. Three weeks and three days post-operatively.

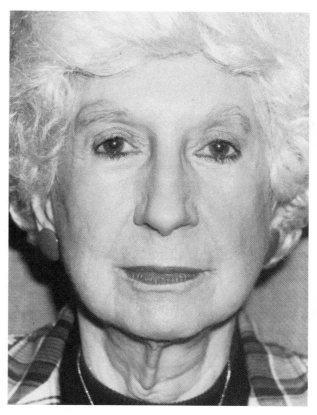

Figure 63h. Resolution and good result with adequate cleaning, six months post-operatively.

14   Post-Chemical Peel Instructions: A Guide for the Patient

The following instructions are based on the authors' experiences with hundreds of chemical face peel patients and are designed to answer practically every question regarding the "do's" and "don't's" following this procedure. The patient and family should read these instructions several times and become thoroughly familiar with them. *Faithful* adherence to these instructions tends to result in the smoothest post-operative course and most favorable healing. Whenever a question arises, one should refer back to this section; more than likely one will find the answer. If still unsure, by all means, the patient should consult his or her physician.

Failure to follow these instructions faithfully can lead to certain complications, which potentially could jeopardize the desired result.

DISCOMFORT

Following the application of the peel solution, there is a stinging pain that lasts for a few seconds. It then temporarily disappears only to return within several minutes. When it returns it persists for six to eight hours, occasionally longer. This type of discomfort can usually be relieved by taking the prescribed pain tablets and by the application of cooled compresses during this time. A convenient way to fashion the compresses is to put crushed ice in a small plastic zip-lock bag, which can be obtained at most grocery stores. The ice compresses should be discontinued after the pain subsides.

After the first night, discomfort should be negligible and can usually be relieved by regular or buffered aspirin. In fact, *aspirin* is the medication of choice for the pain associated with this type of procedure. (If one has had a face lift or eyelid surgery [blepharoplasty], at the same time use nonaspirin medications.)

SWELLING

As informed before surgery, the patient can expect a moderate-to-severe amount of swelling in the areas treated. This will be especially true for the areas around the eyes and lips. This is only temporary.

Swelling reaches its peak by the second or third day and should begin to subside by the fifth or sixth day. The patient can help decrease the amount of swelling by keeping the head elevated about 30 to 40° when reclining and, by staying up (sitting, standing, walking around) as much as possible. Sometimes the prescribed medications may help reduce the swelling, but gravity and time are more reliable.

SKIN APPEARANCE AND CARE

Within 24 to 36 hours, the peeled area resembles a deep sunburn, or blister, and the patient may notice fluid oozing from the skin. This is expected, because, as the superficial layers of skin begin to separate from the deeper layer, serum accumulates between them and the peeled regions are converted to a "water blister."

Approximately 24 hours following the procedure, the patient should begin *gently* washing the peeled area with body temperature tap water. This is most easily accomplished by standing in a shower and using only the finger tips. The patient should not use a wash cloth. This washing must be repeated six times per day. Following each washing, an ointment or cream, which may be specifically prescribed, should be applied to the peeled areas like a light frosting on a cake to act as a moisturizer, prevent dryness and crusting, and promote healing.

While it is very important to avoid sun exposure and to use sunscreen products for the first six months, ordinary sun exposure after that is allowed. It simply takes time for the new skin to toughen or build up a natural resistance to sun and wind.

In the authors' experience, the results have generally been very good. The degree of improvement is not transient, lasting for a period of time measured in years.

PERTINENT FACTS THE PATIENT SHOULD KNOW

1.   Some skins are more favorable than others; fair complexions tend to do better than dark ones. Thick,

tough, more deeply etched or oily skins may require a two-staged approach for the best results (i.e., a second peel or "touching-up" of several areas at a later time). Like painting a roughly textured wall, deep creases may require a "touch-up."

2. Peeling alone is not indicated for treatment of sagging tissues; although the new skin has better elasticity, this requires surgery. The authors have seen additional tightening in the skin in many patients after a peel.

3. The solution stings as it is applied, but this is short-lived—a matter of seconds. Later discomfort can be eased with appropriate medications. Twilight anesthesia is used for full-face peels; therefore, most patients have amnesia regarding their operating room experience.

4. Considerable swelling may occur for a few days; the patient must be emotionally mature enough and be willing to accept this temporary distortion of appearance to achieve the end result desired. It is best to warn family members about this beforehand. For this reason, the authors usually recommend a stay at their clinic apartments during the first week if one is having a full-face peel.

5. The procedure may be performed in the Clinic, but the authors may require a stay close by for several days (usually three to five days for full-face peels.)

6. When instructions are followed, scarring following peeling is rare.

7. When combined with a face lift, segmental peels (around the mouth or lids) can be done the *next morning* following the face lift surgery. In the authors' experience, swelling is less when the peel is performed *after* the face lift dressing has been removed.

8. The peel is considered a surgical procedure; therefore, the risks that apply to surgery must be considered.

9. One should not take any female hormones or birth control pills for approximately six months after a peel. They can lead to changes in skin pigmentation or color.

10. Post-operative care is extremely important in obtaining the best result. The surgeon should give the patient instructions for caring for the new skin.

11. The "new skin" will be much like the skin of a newborn, in that it will take time for it to toughen and be able to tolerate direct sun, wind exposure, and certain skin care products. Because it is new skin, the texture and color will be somewhat different from what has not been peeled. Makeup can generally camouflage any contrast.

Furthermore, peeling (or dermabrasion) will not reduce the size of pores. A pore is the surface opening of an oil gland or hair follicle. Attempts to reduce its size may lead to the development of a "pimple."

Remember, the peel can sometimes produce a dramatic improvement in the texture of the facial skin.

It may be the best treatment available to the facial surgeon to help obtain a fresher, more youthful skin for his or her patients. Certainly, it is not indicated for every patient; therefore, the surgeon should render an opinion as to whether one is a candidate for this procedure.

The patient should never pick at crusts or pieces of skin that do not loosen easily; also, the patient should apply the prescribed ointment or cream to them liberally and they should peel off with time. (Avoid getting softening agents in the eyes.)

At this time in the healing process, new delicate skin is being formed. Premature removal of the crusts may damage this tender new skin and delay healing.

The patient should never wear a shower cap, wig or hairpiece that contacts any area that has been peeled, as this might result in delayed healing and jeopardize an otherwise good result.

During the first seven days, the delicate new skin is undergoing a "toughening up" process. About the 10th to 14th day, most of the crusting should have disappeared and the new skin will appear intensely pink (the lower lid region is usually the last area for crusting to disappear.) At this stage, the softening agents should be applied more sparingly, but gently rubbed in, as one would use any other moisturizing cream.

Except when following these instructions, the patient should keep the fingers or tissues away from the face. Finger tips contain bacteria and oils and have been in contact with soaps, nail care products, and other materials that might irritate the delicate new skin.

Within about 14 days, the patient should be able to use makeup over the peeled areas. The patient should not institute this alone. The surgeon will discuss this during follow-up Clinic visits. Specific recommendations will be made at that time. Although they do not usually cover as well, water-based makeups are more easily removed, and are therefore recommended for the first few days. Makeup is never applied to unhealed areas.

The authors do not recommend any special brands of makeup. The patient should contact the person or facility one regularly uses for their suggestions, but *hypoallergenic* products are advisable in the beginning.

The intense pink color usually fades rapidly after the second week, but some pink color will remain for six to eight weeks, continually decreasing in intensity.

For awhile, the skin usually appears somewhat tense. The finer wrinkles and the deep grooves should also be less evident.

Occasionally small white cysts may appear in the treated areas. They are stopped-up oil glands and usually disappear in two to three weeks without specific treatment. If they persist, contact the surgeon, who can demonstrate a technique to help eliminate them.

Early in the healing process, exposure to heat, cold, wind, or emotional upset (fear, anger, crying, etc.) will cause the skin to temporarily become intensely pink. This is due to increased blood flow or blushing. After about three to four months, this phenomenon should disappear.

"FEVER BLISTERS"

Patients who have had difficulty with recurrent "fever blisters" or "cold sores" may develop an exacerbation of these lesions four or five days post-operatively. If one has *ever* had this problem, one should take Zovirax® 200 mg every 4 hours for at least 7 days. This can be purchased at the drugstore by prescription. If lesions appear, the patient should call the clinic, so that the surgeon can prescribe a special medication to be applied to the affected areas four times per day. The authors feel this helps prevent spreading of the fever blisters, and often relieves some of the discomfort. Although alarming, the authors have yet to see any permanent effects from them.

MEDICATIONS

When discharged from the clinic, the patient should continue with the medicine being taken before surgery. These should be taken as directed until the supply is exhausted; these prescriptions do not need to be refilled. One should continue taking the prescribed vitamins for three weeks post-operatively, and may also be given several new prescriptions at the time of discharge. One of them is for the relief of pain. A sleeping pill may also be prescribed and should not be filled unless one feels the need. Sometimes an antibiotic will be given. If these are prescribed, they should be started immediately upon arrival home or at the clinic apartment, and should be taken until the supply is finished. If one has a history of fever blisters or cold sores, other medications may be prescribed as mentioned in the section on "Fever Blisters."

RESUMING ACTIVITIES

Wearing Eyeglasses

If the area around the nose has been peeled (as in a full-face peel), one should wait two weeks before wearing eyeglasses. The pressure of glasses resting on the skin of the nose, except for very brief periods of time, is to be avoided.

Sun Exposure

The patient should try to avoid either direct or reflected rays of the sun for at least eight weeks, since pigmentation of the peeled areas may result if the new delicate skin is exposed too early. This means that sunning oneself (golfing, fishing, tennis, or similar activities) during the sunny part of the day should be avoided during the initial eight-week period. The peeled areas should be protected for six months by large brimmed hats and a sunscreen product (such as Sundown®, Supershade®, or a similar product). These products must be worn if one is exposed for prolonged periods.

Skin Care

Continued use of skin moisturizers will be the best adjunct in nurturing the new skin and preserving its smooth and soft texture.

Returning to Work and Resuming Social Activities

When these should commence depends upon the amount of public contact, the amount of sun exposure one's job involves, and the degree of redness and swelling that develops. The average patient returns to work or goes out socially about two weeks after the peel; although, depending upon individual circumstances, social exposure can begin as soon as makeup can be worn.

Athletics

Strenuous athletic endeavors should be avoided for the first month. Exposure to extremes of heat, cold, or wind (as in snow skiing or other such outdoor sports) may damage the new skin and should be avoided for six months. Such exposure certainly causes the skin to become pink because of increased blood flow. However, it should subside in a short while if it occurs. One should care for the new skin as carefully as that of a newborn's. Like a baby's skin, it may have a more delicate texture and possibly a different color. It will gradually toughen and tolerate most of the prepeel activities.

POST-OPERATIVE CLINIC VISITS AND ACCOMMODATIONS

The patient will usually be seen in the clinic the day following the peel procedure, and at several intervals for the first week or two. The exact timing of these visits will vary from individual to individual, depending upon the healing process and the extent of the areas peeled. Every attempt should be made to keep these appointments, since it is vitally important that the surgeon closely monitors the healing. If one lives in another city, one should stay in town for the first week after surgery. Depending upon the extent of the areas peeled, the surgeon may request that the patient stays in one of the apartments adjacent to the clinic. Obviously, if small areas are peeled or "touched-up," the patient may be allowed to go directly home.

The patient should remember that swelling, crusting, and redness are expected with *every* chemical face peel. One may be alarmed at the facial appearance for about one week. Time and diligent skin care will help one to obtain a better result.

Close adherence to these instructions is vital to avoiding problems that might jeopardize the desired result.

It is perfectly normal to go through a period of *depression* following this procedure. It may be related to a letdown from the excitement of waiting for surgery, a hangover from the anesthetic, pain and sleeping medications, and the fact that one's appearance is worse, rather than better, during the first week or so. The patient should not be alarmed; it will pass. Every other patient experiences it too.

The patient should notify the physician if he or she has any questions about the instructions or the healing process.

Failure to follow these instructions faithfully can lead to certain complications, which potentially could jeopardize the desired result.

15 Regional Chemexfoliation in Combination With Facial Surgery

Patients undergoing a blepharoplasty or rhytidectomy should understand that neither of these procedures will remove *all* facial wrinkling. It is often necessary to peel the eyelids, lips, forehead, cheeks, or the full face to obtain the more youthful appearance that the patient desires (Figs. 64 to 66).

Many patients require regional peels in conjunction with facial surgery. Those who undergo a blepharoplasty procedure return for a periorbital chemical peel procedure three to six months post-operatively if significant crow's feet or lid wrinkling are present. Similarly, patients who undergo facelift surgery often require a peel in the perioral region to obtain improvement around the mouth. Perioral peeling can be done at the completion of facelift surgery. However, simultaneous peeling over areas that have been undermined is risky and generally ill advised. If the undermined area needs to be peeled, this can be done three to six months *after* facelift or eyelid surgery. Peeling over an undermined area could increase the risk of full-thickness skin loss and lead to hypertrophic scarring.

A full face peel is delayed three to six months after facelift surgery. Perioral and periorbital peels can be done at the completion of a facelift if a blepharoplasty procedure or perioral surgery is not done. The senior author has, in selected cases, dermabraded and peeled deep forehead creases at the completion of a rhytidectomy procedure if a forehead lift was not performed (Figs. 67 to 81).

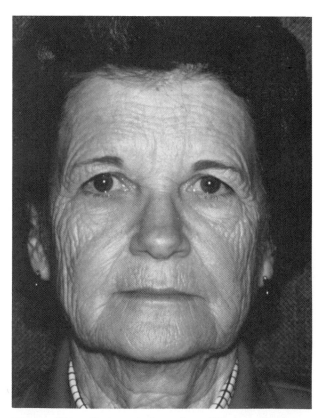

Figure 64a. Patient before face lift and blepharoplasty procedures (antero-posterior view).

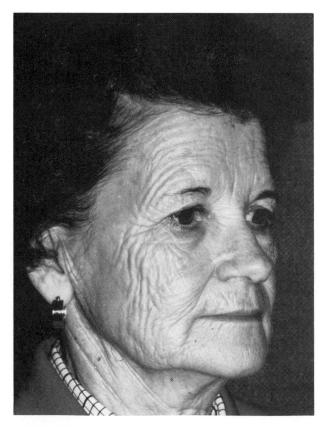

Figure 64b. Oblique view.

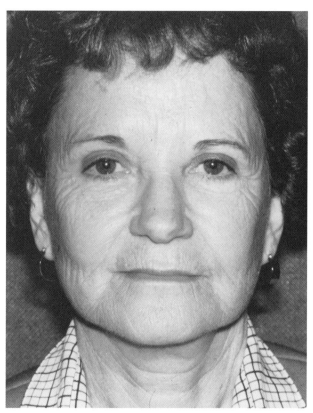

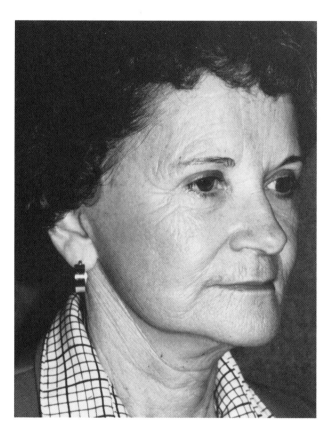

Figure 64c.   Patient after face lift and blepharoplasty procedures and before a chemical peel. Fine wrinkling cannot be removed by a face lift or blepharoplasty (antero-posterior view).

Figure 64d.   Oblique view.

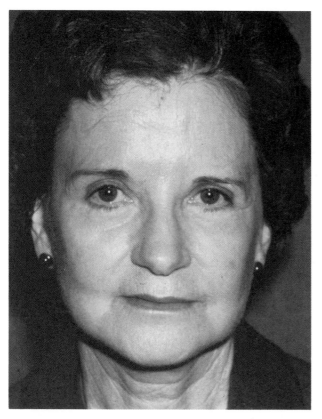

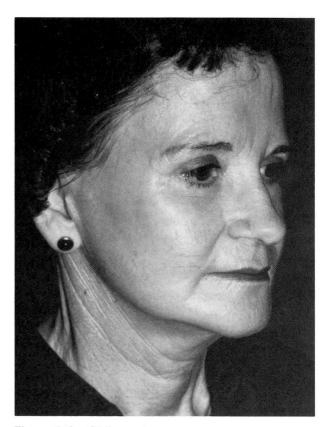

Figure 64e. Post-rejuvenation surgery and chemical peel. Note the improvement in wrinkles (anteroposterior view).

Figure 64f. Oblique view.

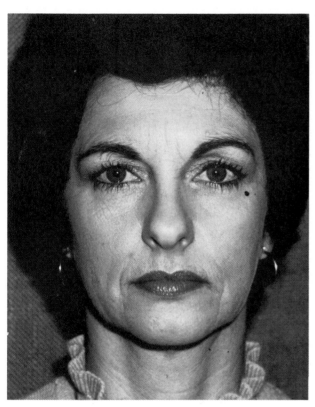 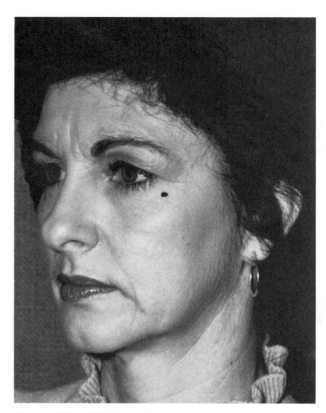

Figure 65a.   Patient before a peel procedure (antero-
posterior view).

Figure 65b.   Oblique view.

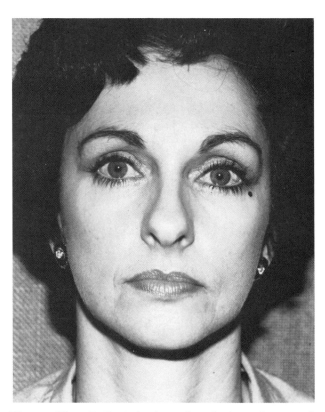 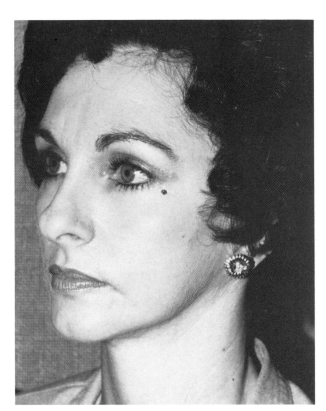

Figure 65c. Patient had a chemical peel several months after a face life and blepharoplasty. Note the improvement in very fine wrinkling of the periorbital region (antero-posterior view).

Figure 65d. Oblique view.

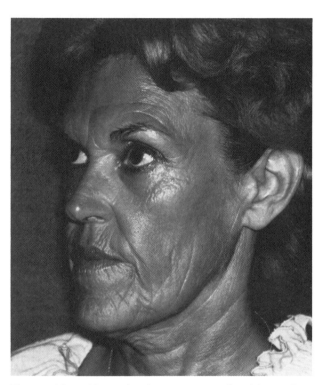

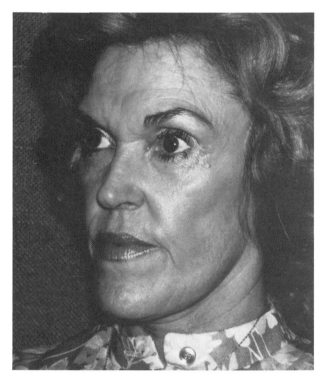

Figure 66a. Note the improvement in this patient with parchment-like skin (pre-operative oblique view).

Figure 66b. Post-operative face lift and blepharoplasty; post-operative chemical peel several months later (oblique view).

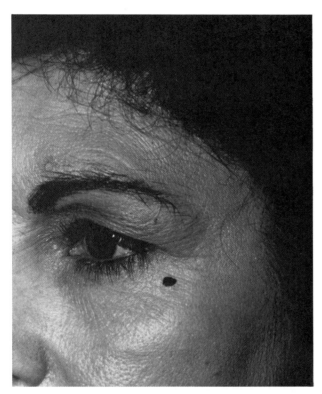

Figure 67a.   Previous patient; pre-operative close-up (periorbital oblique view).

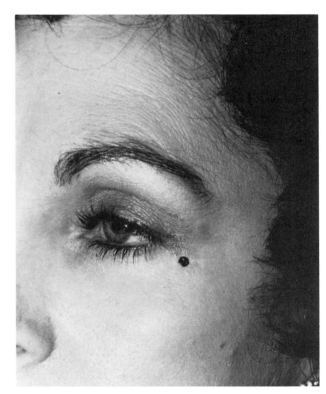

Figure 67b.   Post-operative face lift, blepharoplasty, and chemical peel several months later. Note the improvement with a periorbital peel.

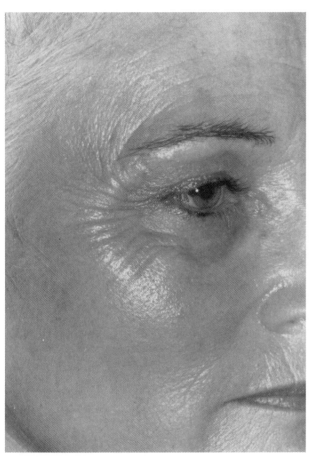

Figure 68a. Pre-operative periorbital chemical peel (periorbital oblique view).

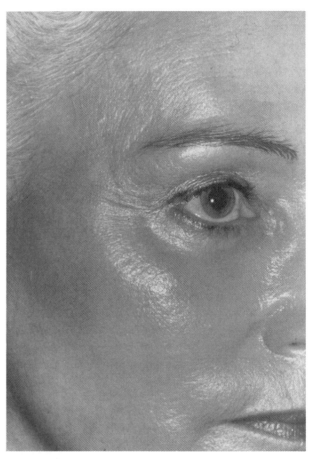

Figure 68b. Note the improvement in crow's feet and upper eyelid skin (periorbital oblique view).

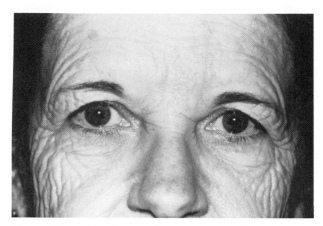

Figure 69a.   Previous patient; pre-operative close-up (periorbital view).

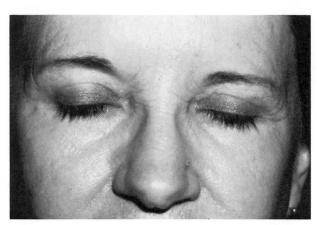

Figure 69d.   Post-operative face lift and blepharoplasty, with a chemical peel, several months later. Note the improvement in periorbital wrinkling. Surgery alone cannot accomplish this type of improvement (close-up periorbital view, eyes closed).

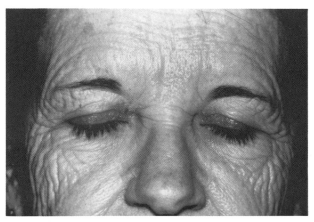

Figure 69b.   Previous patient; pre-operative close-up (periorbital view, eyes closed).

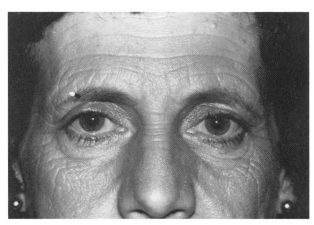

Figure 70a.   Before face lift, blepharoplasty and chemical peel procedures (close-up periorbital view).

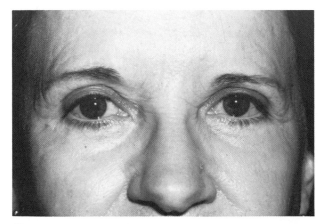

Figure 69c.   Post op facelift, blepharoplasty, with chemical peel, several months later. Note improvement in periorbital wrinkling; Surgery alone cannot accomplish this type of improvement; close-up periorbital view.

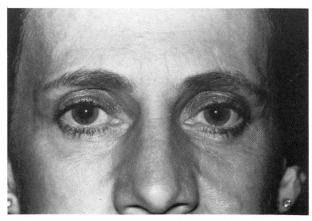

Figure 70b.   Post-surgery and chemical peel. Surgery can remove the excess eyelid tissue and fat herniations, but chemical peeling is responsible for the improvements in wrinkling (close up periorbital view).

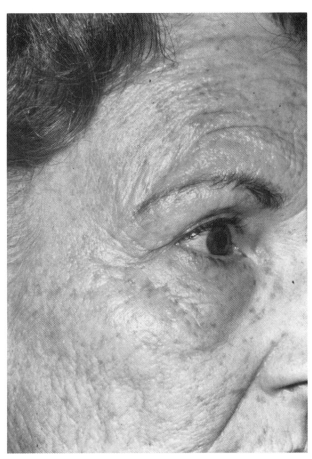

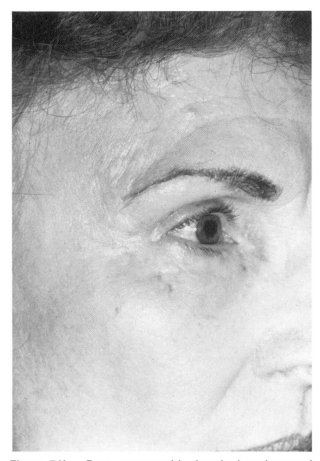

Figure 71a. Before face lift, blepharoplasty, and chemical peel procedures (periorbital oblique view).

Figure 71b. Post-surgery with chemical peel several months later. Surgery is responsible for the reduction in eyelid skin and fat. Note improvement in the wrinkling and pigmentation of the surrounding facial skin, as well as the periorbital skin; a result of the chemical peel (periorbital oblique view).

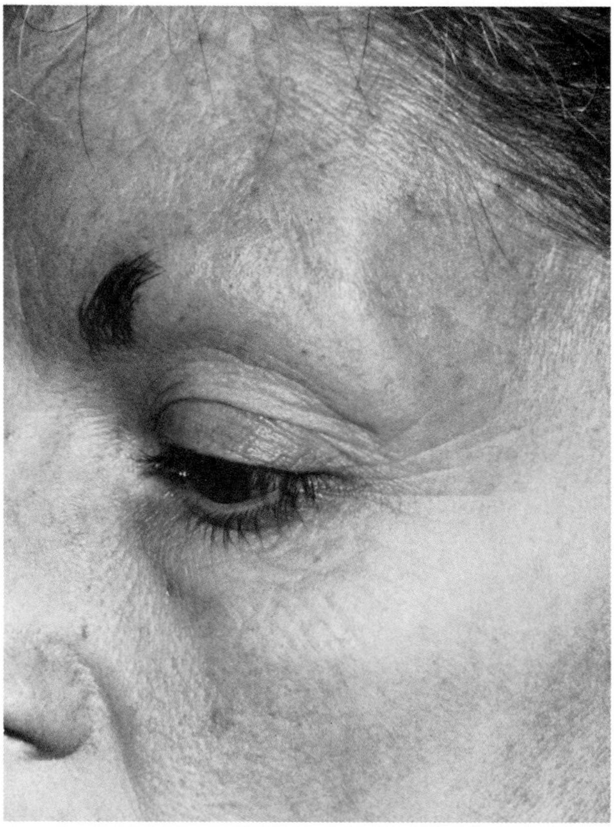

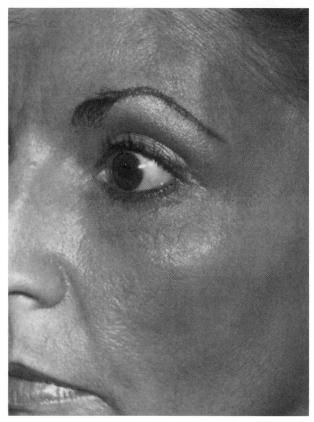

Figure 72a.   Before periorbital chemical peel (periorbital oblique view).

Figure 72b.   Post-operative periorbital chemical peel only. Note the improvement in fine wrinkling (periorbital oblique view).

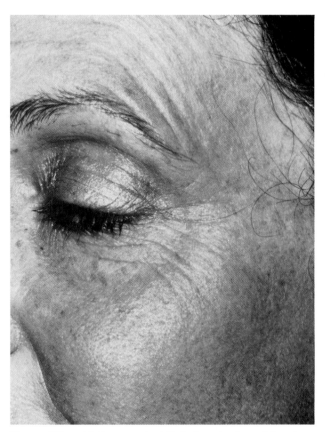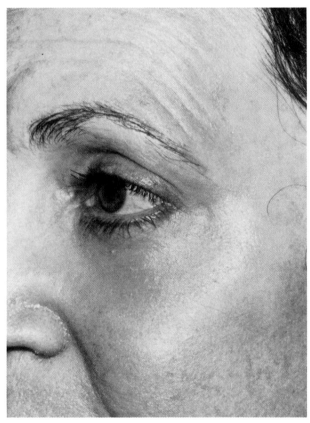

Figure 73a.   Before periorbital chemical peel (periorbital oblique view).

Figure 73b.   Post-operative periorbital chemical peel only. Note the dramatic improvement in periorbital wrinkling (periorbital oblique view).

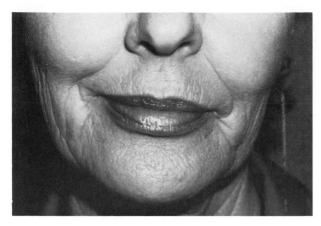

Figure 74a. Before full-face chemical peel (perioral view).

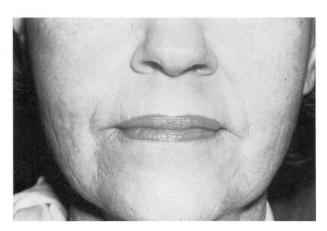

Figure 75b. Improvement in deep perioral wrinkling. Surgery alone will not improve this condition (perioral view).

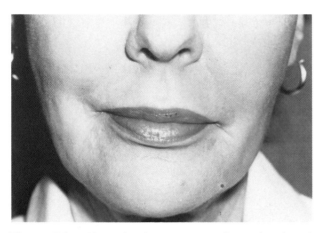

Figure 74b. Note the improvement in perioral and surrounding facial skin wrinkling. No other procedure was performed (perioral view).

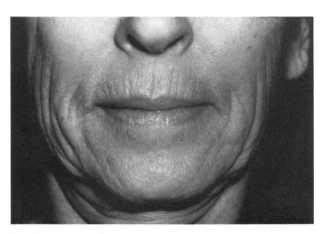

Figure 76a. Before face lift and chemical peel (perioral view).

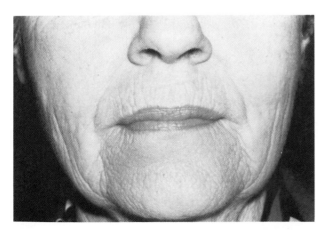

Figure 75a. Before face lift and perioral chemical peel (perioral view).

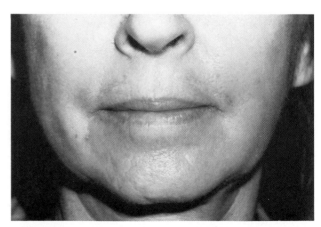

Figure 76b. Post-face lift with chemical peel several months later. Surgery has improved sagging and excess tissue. Chemical peel has improved the fine wrinkling (perioral view).

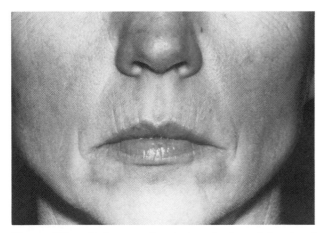

Figure 77a. Before perioral chemical peel (perioral view).

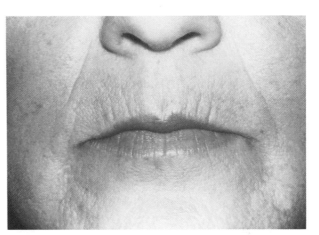

Figure 78a. Before perioral chemical peel (perioral view).

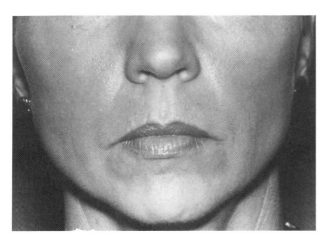

Figure 77b. Improvement in fine wrinkling without surgery (perioral view).

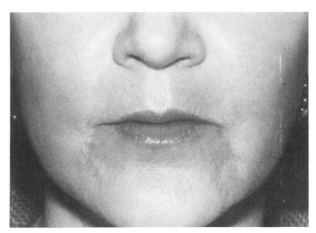

Figure 78b. Excellent improvement in fine wrinkling. Note the improvement in texture of the skin and nasolabial creases. Some wrinkling remains. Contrast difference between the photos is not necessarily the result of exposure discrepancies. Camera exposure and lighting is exactly the same. After peeling, more light reflection may occur in some photographs (perioral view).

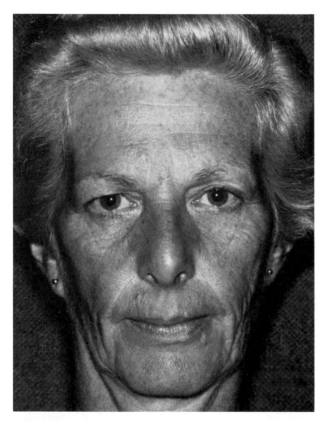

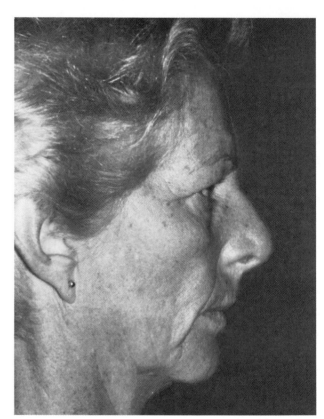

Figure 79a.   Sometimes rejuvenation procedures are substituted with a chemical peel. Not all patients will elect for face lift and blepharoplasty. There may be some tightening or reduction of tissue laxity in some cases. This patient is shown before full-face chemical peel only (antero-posterior view).

Figure 79b.   Lateral view.

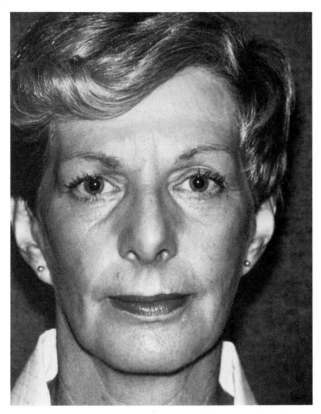

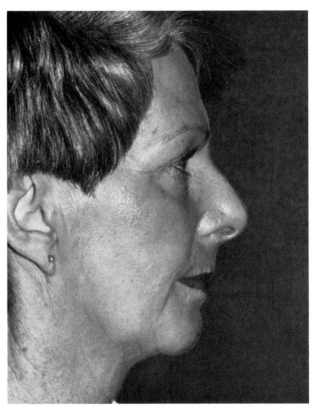

Figure 79c. Note the improvements in all aesthetic units. There is also a reduction in tissue excess along the margin of the mandible, as well as an improvement in the texture of the skin (antero-posterior view).

Figure 79d. Note the reduction of excess tissue along the margin of the mandible, nasolabial fold, and upper eyelid skin (lateral view).

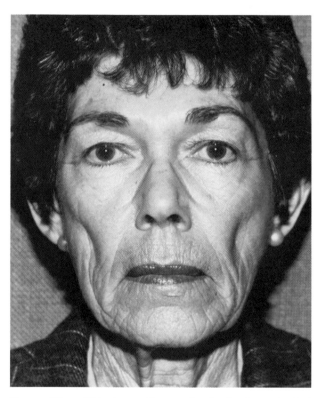

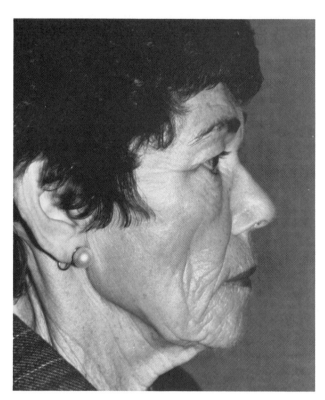

Figure 80a.   This is another patient who has elected for chemical peeling as her only rejuvenation procedure (antero-posterior view).

Figure 80b.   Lateral view.

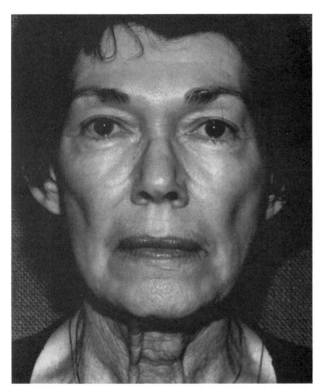

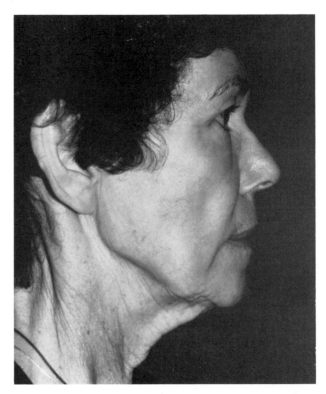

Figure 80c.   There is an overall reduction of wrinkling and some decrease in elasticity. The platysmal banding remains. Surgery would be required to improve this type of excess tissue. The excess upper eyelid tissues are improved, but remain (antero-posterior view).

Figure 80d.   Note again the reduction of wrinkling. The excess tissue along the margin of the mandible and in the neck would require a rhytidectomy (lateral view).

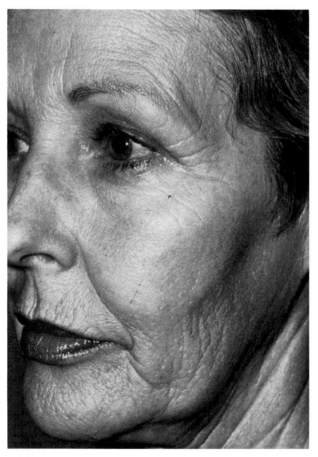

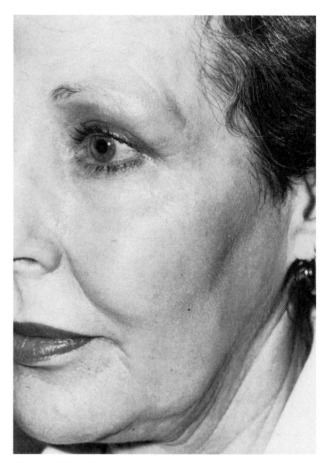

Figure 81a. Before full-face chemical peel only (close-up oblique view).

Figure 81b. Improvements are seen in all aesthetic units. This photograph appears somewhat under-exposed. There is an increase in light reflection post-peel in this patient. However, the apparent improvements are real. There is some decrease in pigmentation (close-up oblique view).

16 Facial Skin Care and Cosmetic Tips: A Guide for the Patient

This chapter will familiarize the patient with some basic facts about enhancing the results of facial plastic surgery by following basic skin care, cosmetic, and grooming tips. It will give one enough background to become an "educated consumer."

Fortunately, during and after the healing process, there are many skin care, cosmetic, and grooming procedures that will promote healing and enhance surgical results. Following these suggestions may help one maintain the positive attitude that is essential to looking one's best.

Women can usually resume cosmetic use about one week after surgery and ten days after dermabrasion or chemical peel. Careful use of makeup can help camouflage bruising and discoloration, and can help one's self-esteem during the healing period.

Water-based cosmetics are usually recommended during the first three weeks, since they can be easily washed off with water if irritation occurs. If the skin is particularly sensitive, one may want to use hypoallergenic makeups. The patient should avoid products that contain fragrance or alcohol during the first few months.

Generally, one can return to one's former makeup routine (including oil-based or perfumed cosmetics) about six weeks after surgery; but many women feel that this is an ideal time to reassess their beauty routine and perhaps make some changes. A consultation with a professional cosmetician can give a real boost.

Incision scars from many facial plastic surgery procedures are hidden and do not present a cosmetic problem. Scars in a noticeable location present problems because they tend to be a different color from surrounding skin, show a texture difference (such as a shiny surface), or they may be slightly raised or lowered.

The first two problems are dealt with by using a foundation makeup with good coverage. Surface irregularities are harder to camouflage because they create shadows that do not mask easily. The patient should avoid trying to cover an irregular scar with makeup. Makeup tends to collect in slight depressions or along the edges of raised scars, making the blemish even more noticeable. Using a sheer foundation and playing up other features to draw the eye away

from the scar may help. It may be possible to use dermabrasion at a later date to even out irregular facial scars.

If regular makeup does not adequately cover bruised or reddened areas, special corrective cosmetics are available. High-coverage makeups have been developed for use by both men and women after plastic surgery, burn or cancer surgery, or to conceal port-wine stains and other severe birthmarks and scars. Such products are available in a variety of shades for all skin tones, including black. Special skin toners or "color block" products are also available in green, pink, and purple to neutralize skin discolorations. Corrective cosmetics and skin toners are available commercially, and can be purchased at most department store cosmetic counters.

MAKEUP TIPS FOR A NATURAL APPEARANCE

• Always select a foundation that is one shade lighter than your natural skin tone.

• Use a translucent powder after foundation for complete coverage with a soft, natural look.

• A concealer (stick or cream) may be applied under the eyes to mask bruises or dark circles. Apply it under your foundation, and use a shade slightly lighter than your base color.

• Use a green skin toner to balance excessive redness, pink to counteract a sallow complexion, and purple to mask yellow discoloration.

• Avoid brown or black eyeliner after eyelid surgery, as these colors tend to emphasize redness. Blue eyeliner, smudged along the lash line on both the upper and lower lids, helps to minimize redness and dark circles.

• Scars in the eyebrow area may leave brow hairs missing. Use a small, angled brush to shade the missing area, using a flat shadow color close to your hair color. This looks more natural than shading with eyebrow pencil.

• A soft eyeshadow pencil in slate or taupe can be smudged toward the outer corner of the eye to correct any visible scars in this area.

• Avoid using metallic or iridescent eyeshadow or face makeup, as these colors emphasize open pores, scars, and other skin flaws.

• After a facelift, choose a soft, faceframing hairdo. Hair that is too short around the face, and hair that is swept up off the forehead may reveal scars. Medium-length bangs, perhaps gently curled, can help to camouflage scars in the forehead area.

• If hairline and forehead scars are not a problem, a soft, full backswept hairstyle can promote a youthful appearance. Avoid severely pulled-back styles.

If you have a reddened complexion or redness around the eyes, never wear fuschia, rose, red, or hot pink. Instead, choose soft shades of blue and green for the wardrobe and makeup.

Bibliography

American Academy of Facial Plastic and Reconstructive Surgery: *Post-Operative Facial Skin Care and Cosmetic Tips,* 1986.

Baker TJ: The ablation of rhytids by chemical means—A preliminary report. *J Florida Med Assoc* 1961;48:451.

Beeson WH, McColough EG: Chemical face peeling without taping. *J Dermatol Surg Oncol* 1985;11(10):985-990.

Burks JW: *Wire Brush Surgery in the Treatment of Certain Cosmetic Defects and Diseases of the Skin.* Springfield, Ill, Charles C Thomas, 1956.

Cortez E: Post peel topical steroid application. Personal communication, Kansas City, Mo, 1987.

Maibach HF, Rovee DT: *Epidermal Wound Healing.* Chicago, Year Book Medical Publishers, Inc, 1972.

McCollough EG, Hillman RA: Chemical face peel. *Otolaryngol Clin North Am* 1980;13(2):353-365.

McCollough EG: *Surgical Anatomy of the Skin and Wound Healing: Otolaryngology.* Hagerstown, Md, Harper & Row, Inc, 1979, vol 4, chap 3.

Monheit G: Contact dermatitis regimen. Personal communication, Birmingham, Ala, 1986.

Wood-Smith D, Rees TD: Chemabrasion and dermabrasion. In *Cosmetic Facial Surgery.* Philadelphia, WB Saunders Co, 1973, pp 213-220.

Index